Probiotic
and Prebiotic
Recipes for Health

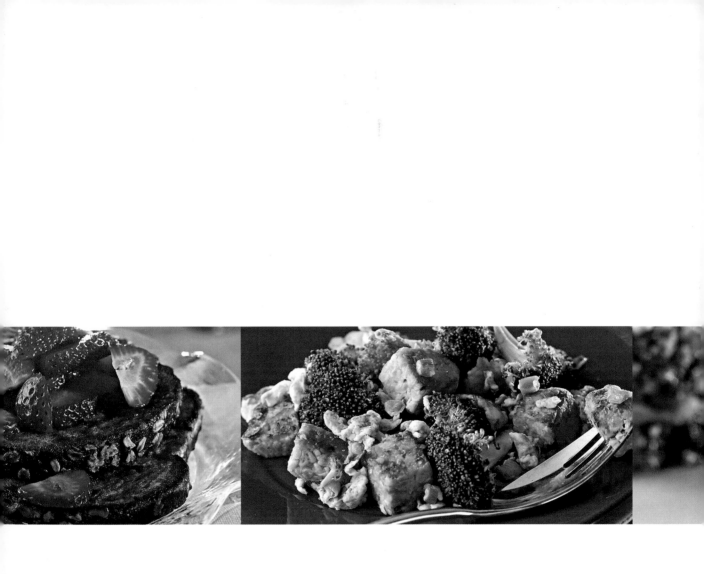

Probiotic and Prebiotic Recipes for Health

100 Recipes That Battle Colitis, Candidiasis, Food Allergies, and Other Digestive Disorders

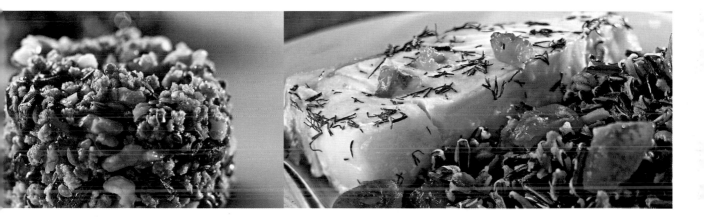

TRACY OLGEATY GENSLER,

M.S., R.D.

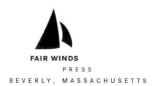

FAIR WINDS

PRESS

BEVERLY, MASSACHUSETTS

Text © 2008 Fair Winds Press

First published in the USA in 2008 by
Fair Winds Press, a member of
Quayside Publishing Group
100 Cummings Center
Suite 406-L
Beverly, Massachusetts 01915-6101
www.fairwindspress.com

12 11 10 09 08   1 2 3 4 5

ISBN-13: 978-1-59233-321-9
ISBN-10: 1-59233-321-4

Library of Congress Cataloging-in-Publication Data
Gensler, Tracy Olgeaty.
    Probiotic and prebiotic recipes for health : 100 recipes that battle colitis,
candidiasis, food allergies, and other digestive disorders / Tracy Olgeaty Gensler.
        p.   cm.
    ISBN-13: 978-1-59233-321-9
    ISBN-10: 1-59233-321-4
    1. Digestive organs—Diseases—Diet therapy—Recipes. 2. Probiotics—Popular works.
3. Prebiotics—Popular works. 4. Colitis—Diet therapy—Recipes. 5. Candidiasis—Diet therapy—Recipes.
6. Food allergy—Diet therapy—Recipes. I. Title.
    RC806.G46 2008
    641.5'631--dc22
                                                                                    2007042325

Book design: Sheila Hart Design, Inc.
Photography: Glenn Scott Photography

Printed and bound in China

I am deeply grateful to the following people for their dedication to this project: Michelle Hering Kennedy, M.S., C.P.T., Amy Anderson, Ph.D. candidate, David A. Mark, Ph.D., Z Altug, M.S., P.T., C.S.C.S.

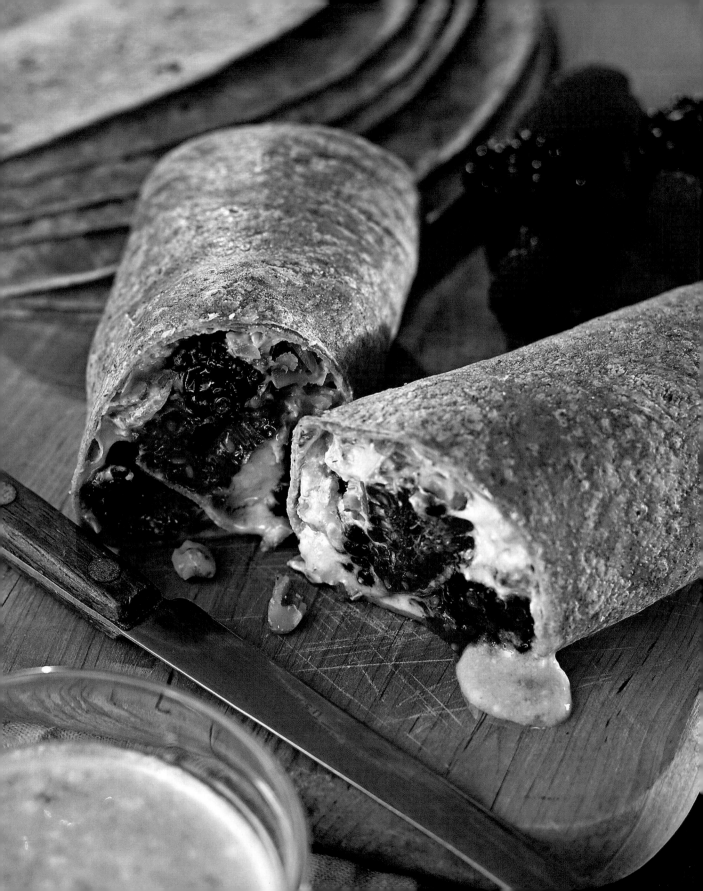

Contents

Introduction

Some people say you are what you eat. And maybe they're right. After all, every bit of bacteria that sets up camp in your digestive system is there because you ate it, drank it, breathed it in, or touched it. It's well established that much of our immunity—our ability to fight the common cold, the stomach flu, and maybe even cancer and a host of other diseases— is linked to the bacteria that harbor in the large intestine. Smoking, gastric bypass surgery, and even drinking alcohol can alter intestinal bacteria, allowing bad bacteria to triumph over the good, leaving you vulnerable to digestive upset and illness.

We seek out opportunities to make dietary changes to improve our chances of staying healthy, missing less work, enjoying vacations, and living well into our retirement years. The Centers for Disease Control and Prevention says, "It's no secret that good nutrition plays an essential role in maintaining health," with campaigns focusing on eating well for the healthiest body weight. The American Heart Association offers diet tips for preventing sudden heart attacks and managing blood cholesterol, blood pressure, and body weight. The USDA Dietary Guidelines include simple, health-promoting guidance that mirrors the probiotic and prebiotic recipes included in this book, which

- emphasize fruits, vegetables, whole grains, and nonfat or low-fat milk and milk products;
- include lean meats, poultry, fish, beans, eggs, and nuts;
- are low in saturated fats, trans fats, cholesterol, salt (sodium), and added sugars.

Eating healthfully for disease prevention is the cry heard around the planet, and functional foods such as probiotics are gaining popularity as people strive to improve their health. Health professionals such as gastroenterologists, nutritionists, and researchers are recommending probiotic and prebiotic foods to help alleviate gastrointestinal symptoms and improve immunity. By choosing a probiotic- and prebiotic-rich diet, the millions of people suffering from irritable bowel syndrome, lactose intolerance, gluten intolerance, and other digestive disorders can get some relief from symptoms such as diarrhea, constipation, gas, bloating, and discomfort.

The research regarding the health benefits of probiotic and prebiotic foods is limited but very promising, with literally hundreds of current studies on the topic. The press is also hot on the probiotics trail, with frequent features on television, in newspapers, and in consumer magazines. In addition to the delicious recipes inside, this book spells it all out for you: how the digestive system works and why the correct balance of bacteria in your digestive tract—encouraged by probiotic and prebiotic foods—leads to better defense against many illnesses. You'll also learn how easy it is to choose probiotic and prebiotic foods from the grocery shelf and the four important questions to ask to make sure the products are right for you. In addition, this book offers suggestions for understanding how to read research studies—an important skill moving forward on your path to optimal health.

While there is growing interest in natural, health-promoting diets, it can be hard to translate this to food selection and preparation. In this book, you'll find easy recipes for weaving probiotic and prebiotic foods into your daily meals. One hundred recipes await: breakfasts, lunches, dinners, and snacks, including delicious dishes such as Waldorf salad (with toasted walnuts and thinly sliced tart green apple over a bed of baby greens, tossed in a creamy yogurt-poppy salad dressing), blackberry smoothie, fresh purple and green cabbage salad topped with sautéed tempeh cubes, and whole-wheat pasta with an olive and garlic marinara sauce. The ingredients are minimal, which makes this book a recipe for success!

CHAPTER ONE

Achieving a Healthy Balance in Your Digestive Tract

Like many of the body's systems, your digestive system is a medical marvel. Digestive juices, enzymes, and bacteria live in your digestive tract and help to digest food. When you're born, your digestive tract is a clean slate with no microbes or bacteria at all, but nature solves this problem right away. The moment you took your first taste of milk and put your thumb in your mouth, both good and bad bacteria started to make their homes in your intestines. Bacteria are microbes that can live just about anywhere. They reproduce often and easily and move about effortlessly via thread-like attachments that look like a tail. The bacteria in your digestive tract are a complex ecosystem harboring about 1,000 micro-organisms composed of nearly 400 bacterium species.

New research shows that a balance of bacteria is critical to overall health, with reported health benefits such as fighting diarrhea and improving your immune function. Good bacteria are vital for development of your immune system. The vast majority of the time, as a result of this well-maintained balance, you don't get sick when you're exposed to illness-causing germs. When the delicate balance of good-versus-bad bacteria is overthrown, however, disease-causing bad bacteria can take over the good bacteria and upset the normal, healthy balance in your gut. Yeasts, fungi, and parasites can also contribute to this unhealthy balance.

Bacteria in your digestive tract also help you digest fiber, which your digestive tract is not otherwise equipped to do. Plant foods that provide these indigestible components are particularly healthful; in a strange turn of events, as your bacteria help to digest fiber from plant foods, the by-products of digestion actually feed your intestinal cells. This keeps your digestive system fueled and running smoothly and is why health professionals around the planet strongly recommend a fiber-rich diet, which will be easy to get with the recipes in this book.

A healthy balance of digestive flora can also help produce lactase, an enzyme that digests the milk sugar lactose. Certain probiotic bacteria help alleviate the symptoms of lactose intolerance, relieve diarrhea and constipation, and treat colitis. Research suggests that maintaining a healthy balance of bacteria through a diet rich in probiotic and prebiotic foods can help you

- increase nutrient bioavailablity (your body's ability to use a nutrient);
- treat food allergies, suppress tumors, and detoxify carcinogens;
- treat rheumatoid arthritis;
- improve urogenital health;
- lower blood cholesterol LDL (low-density lipoproteins) and triglycerides, reducing your risk for heart disease;
- lower blood pressure in people with hypertension;
- reduce risk of colon or bladder cancer;
- prevent or treat atopic dermatitis;
- treat urinary tract infections and candidiasis.

(For details on which prebiotic and probiotic bacterial strains are helpful for each condition, see chapter 3: Relief for Specific Illnesses and Diseases.)

The Culprits

The healthy balance of your digestive tract can be upset by several factors, including antibiotic misuse (see sidebar), a high-fat diet, a diet high in refined sugars, and a high-meat diet. A healthy lifestyle also means not smoking, avoiding intestinal surgery such as gastric bypass, and exercising (see chapter 5: Live Well for Digestive Health). It is possible to create and maintain a healthy balance in your digestive tract, and these recipes will help you achieve optimal digestive bacterial balance with low-fat, low-sugar, meatless, prebiotic, and probiotic foods.

ANTIBIOTIC MISUSE = BUGS GONE WILD

Even though we sometimes need antibiotics to treat a bacterial infection, there's an ugly side to the treatment. Antibiotic overuse and misuse can kill good bacteria along with bad bacteria. A study published in 2005 in the *British Journal of Nutrition* warned that overuse of antibiotics reduced their effectiveness. The study concluded that while they are effective at inhibiting pathogens, antibiotics should not be prescribed in the absence of disease and shouldn't be used for preventive care. Prebiotic and probiotic foods can also inhibit pathogen production, and research shows they can help manage the unpleasant side effects of antibiotic use, including gas, cramping, or diarrhea.

The familiarity people have with antibiotics has given rise to overuse. In a CDC study of over 10,000 people, 28 percent believed that taking antibiotics while they had a cold helped them recover more quickly, and 45 percent said that they *expected* to leave the doctor's office with a prescription for antibiotics when they had a cold, particularly if they were sick enough to visit the doctor. In the cleverly titled campaign "Sniffles or sneeze, no antibiotics please," the Centers for Disease Control and Prevention (CDC) advises parents to stop asking for antibiotics when their children have colds or flu viruses. Such misuse of antibiotic drugs can boost the appearance of drug-resistant, disease-causing bacteria.

A startling development is that almost every type of harmful bacteria has become less responsive to antibiotic treatment, so even if you have a bacterial infection requiring antibiotics, they may not help. The danger is that close contact with coworkers, friends, classmates, and family members can spread this new and more resistant strain of bacteria, making it increasingly difficult to treat. The CDC reports that antibiotic resistance is one of the world's most pressing public health problems.

Diet and Intestinal Health

For years, health professionals have recommended a healthful diet for disease prevention. It's the way you eat over the course of years that contributes to good health, so fad dieting won't get you on the track to optimal intestinal health. Instead, the American Heart Association recommends a diet low in total fat as well as saturated and trans fats to help control blood cholesterol and low-density lipoprotein (LDL) levels. The USDA, meanwhile, recommends limiting refined sugars and using them only as "discretionary calories," which comprise only 100 to 300 calories per day. Its dietary guidelines focus on fruits, vegetables, whole grains, and nonfat or low-fat milk and milk products; include lean meats, poultry, fish, beans, eggs, and nuts; and are low in saturated fats, trans fats, cholesterol, salt (sodium), and added sugars. It may not come as a surprise, but these recommendations are also important for maintaining the health of your digestive tract through a healthy balance of intestinal bacteria.

A poor diet including too much fat, refined sugars, and animal protein can whittle away the viability of probiotic bacteria as it moves through your digestive tract, keeping the bacteria from reaching your large intestine intact, ready to ferment and provide health benefits. Let's take a look at some of the biggest diet offenders:

High-Fat Diet

A high-fat diet can cause an imbalance in the bacteria of the small intestine, causing them to break down the bile salts that are needed to digest and emulsify fats. However, it's important to get your fats straight. While omega-3 fats found in foods such as flaxseed and salmon don't prove harmful for digestive health, it's well established that omega-6 fats and especially saturated and trans fats raise blood cholesterol and are linked to inflammation, heart disease, and possibly even cancer. (See chapter 4: Nutrition for Digestive Health to learn more about foods with good and bad fats.) Trans fats are the biggest threat to your health since they not only raise blood cholesterol, they also lower high-density lipoprotein (HDL) levels, or good cholesterol, which helps protect against heart attacks. Foods that are high in saturated fat are usually high in total fat too—a big problem for digestion.

A high-fat diet also may contribute to colon tumor production and may affect the production of secondary bile acids in the colon. Bile acids are the end product of cholesterol metabolism in the liver and play a role in fat emulsion and detoxification. Colonic luminal bacteria are catalysts in the reaction to produce secondary bile acids, a process that can be interrupted by a diet high in fat.

When intestinal bacteria are out of balance, the fat-soluble vitamins A, D, E, and K aren't well absorbed. This can lead to diarrhea and, eventually, a vitamin A, D, E, or K deficiency. Vitamin D and K deficiency can lead to calcium malabsorption and weakened bones, and vitamin D deficiency is linked to numerous diseases. Vitamin A deficiency, while quite rare, can cause dry eye, night blindness, skin disorders, infections, diarrhea, and respiratory disorders. Vitamin E deficiency, also very rare, can cause muscle weakness, neurological complications, and neuropathy.

High-Meat Diet

A diet high in animal protein can inhibit beneficial bacteria and promote detrimental bacteria. Two kinds of bacteria increase on this type of diet: sulfur-reducing bacteria and 7-alpha-dehydroxylating bacteria.

Fermentation takes place in your colon, feeding healthy bacteria and helping reduce your risk for disease. Too much meat plays havoc with fermentation. A diet high in meat (this includes poultry, cow, pig, game, and organ meats) leads to higher levels of amino compounds, nitrosamines, and changed enzyme patterns, which adversely affect the composition of colonic bacteria.

People following a high animal protein diet have more hydrogen-producing bad bacteria and less methane-producing good bacteria, and this negative balance of bacteria is thought to increase risk for colon cancer. Consider the rate at which African-Americans are diagnosed with colon cancer (60 per 100,000 people) compared to native Africans (1 per 100,000). Native Africans consume very little animal protein (and, surprisingly, not much more fiber than African-Americans). The high-meat diet among African-Americans is thought to be a major factor in the increased incidence of colon cancer.

But will you get enough protein with these meatless recipes? Rest assured that these dishes provide all of the protein you need from nonfat and low-fat milk, low-fat cheese, eggs, and beans.

High-Sugar Diet

You'll find naturally occurring sugars in your prebiotic and probiotic recipes, but you won't find too much refined sugar. That's because simple sugars don't properly nourish the environment in your digestive tract for optimal bacterial growth. A 1999 animal study in the *Journal of Applied Microbiology* examined intestinal bacteria on two different diets: a high-sucrose diet and a diet high in corn starch (a complex carbohydrate). The sucrose diet led to a 12 percent reduction in good bacteria, specifically *clostridium* and *propionibacterium*, when compared to the corn starch diet.

The Vitamin Connection

Your intestinal bacteria have another very important job. They produce enzymes that help you digest hormones and drugs, and they communicate with your liver to produce more enzymes as needed. When good and bad bacteria are out of balance, vitamins aren't properly absorbed. Good bacteria are critical for producing vitamin K as well as thiamin, riboflavin, vitamin B12, and biotin. Here is an outline of the function and deficiency symptoms of most of these important vitamins; more information on vitamin B12 is on pp 66–68 ("Vitamin B12— A Special Vitamin").

Vitamin	Function	Deficiency Symptoms
Vitamin K	Essential for the function of proteins involved in blood clotting, bone mineralization, and cell growth	Problems with blood clotting and increased bleeding, sometimes seen as nosebleeds; blood in urine and stool and heavy menstrual bleeding
Thiamin (Vitamin B1)	Needed for nervous system and muscle functioning; flow of electrolytes in and out of cells; enzyme processes involving thiamin pyrophosphate, carbohydrate metabolism, and HCL (hydrochloric acid) production for proper digestion	This water-soluble, B-complex vitamin is not easily stored in the body. Depletion can happen in as little as fourteen days. Chronic, severe thiamin deficiency (beriberi) can result in potentially serious complications involving the digestive, nervous, or muscular system
Riboflavin	Small amounts of riboflavin are present in most human tissues. It's important for energy production, growth, and cell function	Anemia, glossitis (tongue swelling), throat swelling, throat soreness, weakness, cheilosis/angular stomatitis (skin cracking, sores at the corners of the mouth), dermatitis
Biotin	Important for fatty-acid formation, glucose formation, and their uses as energy sources for the body; metabolism of amino acids and carbohydrates	Skin rash, loss of hair, high blood cholesterol, heart problems

Functional Foods

Functional foods are defined as foods containing some component that affects a function in the body, in a targeted way, to promote healthfulness. Prebiotics and probiotics are functional foods that are proven to enhance many digestive functions, and you can get all of the bacteria you need by eating both prebiotic- and probiotic-rich foods. The benefits of these foods include a controlled transit time in the digestive tract, which improves absorption of nutrients, and improvement in bowel habits and mucosal motility (to promote bowel regularity). Prebiotic and probiotic foods also show great promise for modifying gastrointestinal immune activity.

Prebiotic foods are non-digestible, carbohydrate rich food ingredients (specifically, oligosaccharides—such as inulin—and oligofructose) that are thought to decrease blood cholesterol, LDL, and triglycerides. Triglycerides are blood fats which, when elevated, are strongly connected with coronary artery disease. Because they aren't absorbed in the upper part of the digestive tract, prebiotic foods can make their way to the colon, stimulating good bacteria to grow and altering the microflora in the colon to a healthy composition.

The live microbes in probiotic foods can be used in conjunction with prebiotics, and this combination, synbiotics, can improve the survival of probiotics in the digestive tract.

Although these recipes don't focus on specialized synbiotic action, some of the recipes do include both prebiotic and probiotic foods, and this is an interesting area of research that should be followed closely.

The research on health benefits is fairly new; it's interesting to note that prebiotics were originally thought to impair the absorption of minerals, which are bound in the small intestine. But now, even though the binding action is not disputed, prebiotics are thought to instead *facilitate* the absorption of calcium and magnesium from the colon.

You'll find tasty, easy ways to prepare prebiotic and probiotic foods in these recipes. But first, let's take a look at what happens to the foods you eat during digestion and how this affects bacterial action.

PROBIOTIC AND PREBIOTIC FOODS

Probiotic foods include buttermilk, kefir, kimchi (Korean fermented cabbage), miso, sauerkraut, tempeh (fermented soy), and yogurt.

Prebiotic foods include barley; flax; legumes such as black beans, chickpeas, kidney beans, lentils, navy beans, and white beans; oatmeal; and *all* fruits and vegetables—but especially bananas, berries, chard, collard greens, dandelion greens, garlic, kale, leeks, mustard greens, onions, and spinach.

YOUR DIGESTION: WHO'S IN CHARGE?

A fascinating feature of the digestive system is that it contains its own regulators. The major hormones that control the functions of the digestive system are produced and released by cells in the mucosa of the stomach and small intestine. These hormones are released into the blood of the digestive tract, travel back to the heart and through the arteries, and eventually return to the digestive system, where they stimulate digestive juices and cause peristalsis. Peristalsis, the smooth muscle contractions that move food through the digestive tract, is controlled by the autonomic nervous system (ANS). A bacterial imbalance can disrupt this process by adversely affecting the ANS. The hormones that control digestion are gastrin, secretin, and cholecystokinin (CCK); additional hormones including ghrelin and peptide YY in the digestive system regulate appetite and the intake of food for energy.

A well-regulated digestive system will allow the prebiotic and probiotic bacteria you eat to move through these stages untouched until they reach the large intestine. By the time food reaches the large intestine, or colon, digestive hormones and juices are no longer secreted because digestion is complete.

Hormone	Function	Bacterial Action
Gastrin	Causes the stomach to produce an acid for dissolving and digesting some foods. It is necessary for the normal growth of the lining of the stomach, small intestine, and colon.	Gastrin can penetrate the mucous lining of the stomach or duodenum. This may result in an ulcer because gastrin is able to reach the stomach lining via *Heliobacter pylori* (*H. pylori*), a bad bacterium. *H. pylori* can thrive in the acid environment of the stomach. Probiotics alleviate the symptoms of the *H. pylori* ulcer, but in some cases *H. pylori* needs to be treated with antibiotics.
Secretin	Causes the pancreas to send out a digestive juice that is rich in bicarbonate. It stimulates the stomach to produce pepsin, an enzyme that digests protein, and it also stimulates the liver to produce bile.	Secretin is thought to influence *H. pylori* action as well.
CCK (cholecystokinin)	Causes the pancreas to grow and produce the enzymes of pancreatic juice, and it causes the gallbladder to empty.	Some animal studies show that CCK increases motility of contents through the small intestine and reduces the chance for intestinal bacterial overgrowth. This overgrowth can lead to an imbalance of bad over good bacteria.
Ghrelin	Is produced in the stomach and upper intestine, in the absence of food in the digestive system, to stimulate appetite.	Ghrelin production may be impaired by *H. pylori*. It is thought that the presence of this bacteria decreases the blood concentration of ghrelin, and this in turn decreases appetite, which can lead to reduced and selective food intake (in other words, you may not make healthful choices).
Peptide YY	Is produced in the GI tract in response to a meal in the system, and inhibits appetite.	Animal studies show that too much peptide YY can be stimulated as a result of a high-fat diet. This can, in turn, cause constipation (slow intestinal transit time), which can throw off the balance of good and bad bacteria.

Reprinted with permission from the National Institute of Diabetes and Digestive and Kidney Diseases, U.S. Department of Health and Human Services, 2007.

The Anatomy of Digestion

Every time you eat and drink, you introduce bacteria to your digestive tract. Hormones help move the digestive process along and maintain bacterial balance in your colon. From your mouth to your colon, food and drink must be changed into smaller molecules of nutrients in order for your body to use them as nourishment.

Starting at your mouth, this system is a series of tube-like organs that go through your body. Your digestive system is lined with mucosa and very small glands that secrete juices to help you digest food and liquids. The good bacteria, such as those in prebiotic and probiotic foods, have to make their way through your system all the way to your colon to improve immunity and fight disease there. But both bad bacteria and good bacteria can potentially be killed in the stomach and the small intestine. Envision each bite of food or gulp of liquid hopping on a train in your mouth. Digestion takes place in small steps on the train; first in your mouth, then in your stomach and small intestine, with the glands producing different digestive enzymes at each stop along the way. Some of the digestive juices are produced by the liver and the pancreas, and your nerves and bloodstream also play a major role in digestion.

The Mouth

Digestion actually begins when you put food or drink in your mouth and mastication (a fancy word for chewing) occurs. A little carbohydrate digestion starts here, and a bit of triglyceride breakdown also begins with an enzyme secreted in the mouth but activated in the stomach by chloride ions. Probiotic bacteria survive this first step along the digestive process.

The Stomach

In the lower stomach, food is churned by peristaltic waves that propel the mixture (known as acid-chyme) against the muscle (the pyloric sphincter) at the base of the stomach as it enters the small intestine. It takes one to two hours for the stomach to empty. The nutrient content of your food impacts what happens in your stomach. If you've ever had a stomachache after eating a bucket of french fries or a rack of ribs, it's because a high-fat diet takes longer to digest, and this can feel heavy and uncomfortable.

Your stomach acid may prove to be a hostile environment for the probiotic bacteria as well as the bad bacteria you ingest. According to a 2001 study published in the *American Journal of Clinical Nutrition*, "Before reaching the intestinal tract, probiotic bacteria must first survive transit through the stomach." The secretion of gastric acid there creates a hostile environment for both good and bad bacteria. So how do you protect the good probiotic bacteria? The type and the number of bacteria you eat are important factors in whether enough of them can reach the large intestine and provide a health benefit. (See p 30: "Survival of the Fittest Bacteria.")

The Small Intestine

The main site for digestion and absorption of nutrients, the small intestine, begins with the duodenum. The liver and pancreas secrete hormones and enzymes to aid with digestion here, and the epithelial cells in the duodenum get into the action with a secretion of watery mucous. Carbohydrate and protein digestion continues, and fats are completely digested in the small intestine. Bile salts here mix with the chyme, and these salts have a bactericidal effect, killing some strains of probiotic bacteria along with the bad bacteria.

The inside surface of the small intestine has circular folds that increase the area for absorption, nearly tripling the surface area. Little finger-like structures covered in epithelial cells called villi line the inside of the intestine, increasing the surface area again by tenfold. And since your small intestine is clearly making the biggest effort to snare every possible nutrient, the villi are *also* lined with microvilli, increasing the surface area yet again. These microvilli are formed on top of an epithelial cell known as the brush border.

The cells in the small intestine house lactase, the enzyme used to help digest the milk sugar lactose. Lactase is naturally occurring, but some people lack this enzyme. Eating foods with probiotic bacteria such as *L. acidophilus* and *Bifidobacteria* can help you digest lactose. Kefir, which contains probiotic bacteria as well as inulin, a prebiotic to feed the bacteria, helps to digest lactose as well. Cells in the small intestine also absorb peptide fragments and amino acids across the epithelial cells by a process called active transport.

The small intestine is where people with gluten intolerance run into problems. They are unable to absorb gluten, a protein found in wheat. But there is good news for those suffering from gluten intolerance: Probiotics are currently being tested as a food processing additive that produces pre-digested gliadins for gluten-free foods, increasing the palatability and tolerance of these foods.

The Colon

The large intestine, or colon, is the last stop on the digestion trail. This is where water and electrolytes are recovered and absorbed. The feces are prepared here as well. They are dehydrated and mixed with bacteria and mucous as they get ready to leave the body. This hotspot for bacterial action is moved along by fermentation. If everything has gone as planned, your probiotic bacteria have arrived safely.

We can't understate the benefit of fermentation in the colon; this is the crux of prebiotic and probiotic action in the digestive tract. Both prebiotics and probiotics are very active in the intestinal tract (mainly in the colon) as they maintain a healthy representation of microflora. This healthy balance influences a protective mechanism. In 1993, the *Scandanavian Journal of Gastroenterology* reported that carbohydrate fermentation in the colon is probably the key factor in the prevention of colon cancer. Other studies show benefits of colonic fermentation including improved blood sugar management and blood cholesterol control. Here's how this works: As your colonic contents ferment, prebiotics stimulate the growth of apathogen bacteria, or good bacteria, and increase the short-chain fatty-acid concentration. Short-chain fatty acids are necessary substrates for a healthy gut.

It has been well established that the cells in the colon can elicit immune responses. Probiotics inhibit the growth of pathogen bacteria, or bad bacteria, and help to modulate the intestinal immune system. A 2003 study in the *American Journal of Clinical Nutrition* showed that it's likely the immune benefits are due to more than one probiotic bacterial strain, and it's unlikely that a single probiotic bacterial strain will be capable of influencing the microbial balance in the colon that is necessary for this immune enhancement. Thus, the recipes here include a variety of probiotic bacteria.

Later on, we'll look more closely at the current research regarding prebiotic foods, probiotic microbes, and disease prevention. Some of the beneficial aspects of prebiotic and probiotic foods are still under study, and we can't yet embrace one probiotic bacterial strain as the most beneficial one. Yet as we look at the important actions of good intestinal bacteria, it's hard not to imagine the tremendous potential that prebiotic and probiotic foods have for the body.

CHAPTER TWO

Understanding Probiotics and Prebiotics on the Shelf

It's easier than ever before to find foods that are supplemented with probiotic and prebiotic ingredients. These include the familiar yogurt products, as well as cottage cheese, granola bars, candy bars, frozen yogurt, cookies, and cereal products. Functional foods may be marketed in a few different formats. You might see probiotics and prebiotics packaged as

- supplements, including powders, pills, or liquids

- drugs that are meant to cure, mitigate, or prevent disease
- additives fed to animals that produce the foods ("direct-fed microbials")
- general foods.

Sometimes, small amounts of probiotic bacteria are added to foods and labeled as such, but these don't have a track record for improving health. You need to consume an adequate level of live probiotic bacteria to take advantage of the reported health

Some Yogurts with Live & Active Cultures

Manufacturer	Product Name	Flavors
YoCream International	Original Frozen Yogurt	Original Tart Frozen Yogurt
YoCream International	Nonfat Frozen Yogurt	Nonfat Alpine Vanilla, Nonfat Blueberry Burst, Nonfat Butter Brickle, Nonfat Cappuccino, Nonfat Chocolate Classic, Nonfat Country Vanilla, Nonfat English Toffee, Nonfat Georgia Peach, Nonfat Island Banana, Nonfat Luscious Lemon, Nonfat Outrageous Orange, Nonfat Peppermint Stick, Nonfat Pistachio, Nonfat Pumpkin, Nonfat Very Raspberry, Nonfat White Chocolate Macadamia, Nonfat Apple Spice, Nonfat Boysenberry, Nonfat Cable Car Chocolate, Nonfat Cherry Almond, Nonfat Chocolate Mint, Nonfat Eggnog, Nonfat Fancy French Vanilla, Nonfat Irish Mint, Nonfat Kahlua, Nonfat New York Cheesecake, Nonfat Pecan Praline, Nonfat Pina Colada, Nonfat Plain, Nonfat Root Beer Float, Nonfat Very Strawberry, YoFree Blueberry Nonfat, YoFree Chocolate, YoFree Strawberry Nonfat, YoFree Vanilla Nonfat, YoFree Café au Lait Nonfat, YoFree Raspberry Nonfat, YoFree Strawberry-Banana Nonfat, YoCream Premium Cheesecake Supreme, YoCream Premium French Vanilla, YoCream Premium Natural, YoCream Premium Praline 'n Cream, YoCream Premium Dutch Chocolate, YoCream Premium Milk Chocolate, YoCream Peanut Butter, YoCream Premium White Vanilla

Manufacturer	Product Name	Flavors
YoCream International	YoCream No Sugar Added Yogurt	YoFree Blueberry Nonfat, YoFree Chocolate, YoFree Strawberry Nonfat, YoFree Vanilla Nonfat, YoFree Café au Lait Nonfat, YoFree Raspberry Nonfat, YoFree Strawberry-Banana Nonfat
YoCream International	YoCream Premium	YoCream Premium Cheesecake Supreme, YoCream Premium French Vanilla, YoCream Premium Natural, YoCream Premium Praline 'n Cream, YoCream Premium Dutch Chocolate, YoCream Premium Milk Chocolate, YoCream Premium Peanut Butter, YoCream Premium White Vanilla
Red Mango	Frozen Yogurt	Nonfat Original Frozen Yogurt
Colombo	Colombo Classics	Banana Strawberry, Black Cherry Parfait, Blackberry Burst, Blueberry, Cherry, Peach, Raspberry, Strawberry, Vanilla, White Chocolate Raspberry
Colombo	Colombo Fat Free	Plain, Vanilla
Colombo	Colombo Light Yogurt	Light Blueberry, Light Boston Cream Pie, Light Cherry Vanilla, Light Creamy Vanilla, Light Juicy Peach, Light Key Lime Pie, Light Lemon Meringue, Light Mixed Berry, Light Orange Crème, Light Red Raspberry, Light Strawberry, Light Strawberry Banana
Colombo	Lowfat Yogurt	Lowfat Plain, Lowfat Strawberry, Lowfat Vanilla
Yoplait	GoGurt Portable Yogurt	Strawberry Milkshake, Banana Split, Burstin' Melon Berry, Cool Cotton Candy, Shaggy's Like Cool Punch, Rawberry, Strawberry-Kiwi Kick, Chill-Out Cherry, Strawberry Splash, Berry Blue Blast, Watermelon Meltdown, Strawberry-Banana Burst
Yoplait	Yoplait Kids	Vanilla, Banana, Peach, Strawberry Banana, Strawberry Vanilla, Strawberry
Yoplait	GoGurt Drinks	Red Raspberry, Paradise Punch

benefits—meaning they need to be alive when you consume the food. Transit time, storage, preparation, and expiration date are all factors in how much live bacteria is left when you sit down to eat.

All yogurts made in the United States (this applies to every yogurt, not just the probiotic supplemented yogurts listed on the next page) are made with the probiotic "starter" bacteria *S. thermophilus* and *L. bulgaricus*. Check your yogurt label for the "Live & Active Cultures" seal. This means that the yogurt was not heat-treated after production, and the yogurt should have live versions of these bacteria, even though you still won't know how much live bacteria is in the yogurt at the time you decide to eat it. But don't let this stop you from choosing the foods.

A Sample of Probiotic- and Prebiotic-Enhanced Foods Available in the United States

Manufacturer	Product Name	Type of Probiotic/Prebiotic	Flavors
Kraft	Liveactive Cottage Cheese	Inulin, a natural substance derived from chicory root	Plain, Pineapple, Mixed Berry
Dannon	Activia Yogurt	*Bifidus regularis, Bifidobacterium animalis* DN173010	Strawberry, Peach, Vanilla
Dannon	DanActive Yogurt	*L. casei immunitas*	Strawberry, Cranberry/Raspberry, Vanilla, Blueberry, and Plain
Lifeway	Original Kefir	*Lactobacillus lactis, Lactobacillus rhamnosus, Streptococcus diacetylactis, Lactobacillus plantarum, Lactobacillus casei, Saccharomyces florentinus, Leuconostoc cremoris, Bifidobacterium longum, Bifidobacterium breve, Lactobacillus acidophilus*	Plain
Lifeway	Low Fat Kefir	*Lactobacillus lactis, Lactobacillus rhamnosus, Streptococcus diacetylactis, Lactobacillus plantarum, Lactobacillus casei, Saccharomyces florentinus, Leuconostoc cremoris, Bifidobacterium longum, Bifidobacterium breve, Lactobacillus acidophilus*	Plain, Vanilla, Peach, Strawberries 'n Cream, Raspberry, Strawberry, Banana Strawberry, Cherry, Cappuccino, Blueberry, Pomegranate
Lifeway	Nonfat Kefir	*Lactobacillus lactis, Lactobacillus rhamnosus, Streptococcus diacetylactis, Lactobacillus plantarum, Lactobacillus casei, Saccharomyces florentinus, Leuconostoc cremoris, Bifidobacterium longum, Bifidobacterium breve, Lactobacillus acidophilus*	Plain, Strawberry, Strawberry-Banana, Peach, Raspberry, Blueberry
Lifeway	Organic Whole Milk	*Lactobacillus lactis, Lactobacillus rhamnosus, Streptococcus diacetylactis, Lactobacillus plantarum, Lactobacillus casei, Saccharomyces florentinus, Leuconostoc remoris, Bifidobacterium longum, Bifidobacterium breve, Lactobacillus acidophilus*	Plain, Strawberries and Crème, Wildberries

Nutrition Facts

All flavors: 90 calories, 2 g fat, 1.5 g saturated fat, 15 mg cholesterol, 380 mg sodium, 8 g carbohydrate, 3 g fiber, 4 g sugar, 10 g protein, 150 mg calcium

Strawberry: 110 calories, 2 g fat, 1 g saturated fat, 5 mg cholesterol, 75 mg sodium, 19 g carbohydrate, 0 g fiber, 17 g sugar, 5 g protein, 150 mg calcium
Vanilla: 110 calories, 2 g fat, 1.5 g saturated fat, 10 mg cholesterol, 70 mg sodium, 19 g carbohydrate, 0 g fiber, 17 g sugar, 5 g protein, 150 mg calcium
Peach: 110 calories, 2 g fat, 1 g saturated fat, 10 mg cholesterol, 70 mg sodium, 19 g carbohydrate, 0 g fiber, 17 g sugar, 5 g protein, 150 mg calcium

Strawberry and Cranberry/Raspberry: 90 calories, 1.5 g fat, 1 g saturated fat, 5 mg cholesterol, 45 mg sodium, 17 g carbohydrate, 0 g fiber, 17 g sugar, 3 g protein, 100 mg calcium
Vanilla and Blueberry: 90 calories, 1.5 g fat, 1 g saturated fat, 5 mg cholesterol, 40 mg sodium, 17 g carbohydrate, 0 g fiber, 17 g sugar, 3 g protein, 100 mg calcium
Plain: 90 calories, 2 g fat, 1.5 g saturated fat, 5 mg cholesterol, 40 mg sodium, 15 g carbohydrate, 0 g fiber, 15 g sugar, 3 g protein, 100 mg calcium

162 calories, 8 g fat, 5 g saturated fat, 30 mg cholesterol, 125 mg sodium, 15 g carbohydrate, 3 g fiber, 12 g sugar, 8 g protein, 30 mg calcium

Plain: 120 calories, 2 g fat, 1.5 g saturated fat, 10 mg cholesterol, 125 mg sodium, 12 g carbohydrate, 3 g fiber, 8 g sugar, 14 g protein, 300 mg calcium, 50 IU vitamin D
All other flavors: 174 calories, 2 g fat, 1.5 g saturated fat, 10 mg cholesterol, 125 mg sodium, 25 g carbohydrate, 3 g fiber, 21 g sugar, 14 g protein, 300 mg calcium, 50 IU vitamin D

Plain: 116 calories, 0 g fat, 0 g saturated fat, 5 mg cholesterol, 120 mg sodium, 15 g carbohydrate, 3 g fiber, 12 g sugar, 14 g protein, 300 mg calcium, 50 IU vitamin D
All fruit flavors: 188 calories, 0 g fat, 0 g saturated fat, 5 mg cholesterol, 125 mg sodium, 33 g carbohydrate, 3 g fiber, 30 g sugar, 14 g protein, 300 mg calcium, 50 IU vitamin D

Plain: 160 calories, 8 g fat, 5 g saturated fat, 30 mg cholesterol, 125 mg sodium, 12 g carbohydrate, 3 g fiber, 8 g sugar, 10 g protein, 300 mg calcium
Strawberries and Crème: 212 calories, 8 g fat, 5 g saturated fat, 30 mg cholesterol, 125 mg sodium, 25 g carbohydrate, 3 g fiber, 21 g sugar, 10 g protein, 300 mg calcium
Wildberries: 160 calories, 8 g fat, 5 g saturated fat, 30 mg cholesterol, 125 mg sodium, 25 g carbohydrate, 3 g fiber, 21 g sugar, 10 g protein, 300 mg calcium

A Sample of Probiotic- and Prebiotic-Enhanced Foods Available in the United States—cont'd

Manufacturer	Product Name	Type of Probiotic/Prebiotic	Flavors
Lifeway	Low-fat Organic Kefir	*Lactobacillus lactis, Lactobacillus rhamnosus, Streptococcus diacetylactis, Lactobacillus plantarum, Lactobacillus casei, Saccharomyces florentinus, Leuconostoc cremoris, Bifidobacterium longum, Bifidobacterium breve, Lactobacillus acidophilus*	Plain, Peach, Raspberry, Strawberry
Attune	Wellness Bars	Inulin, *Lactobacillus acidophilus, Lactobacillus casei, Bifiobacterium lactis*	Chocolate Crisp, Cool Mint Chocolate, Blueberry Vanilla, Yogurt and Granola Strawberry Bliss, Yogurt and Granola Wild Berry, and Yogurt and Granola Lemon Crème
Kashi	Vive Cereal	*Lactobacillus* probiotic cultures (*L. acidophilus* or *L. casei*)	Kashi Vive
Horizon Organic	Cottage Cheese	*L. acidophilus, Bifidobacterium*	Regular and Low-Fat
Horizon Organic	Smoothies	*L. acidophilus, Bifidobacterium lactis, S. thermophilus, L. casei*	Strawberry Banana Splash, Wild Berry Blast, Tropical Punch
Horizon Organic	Sour Cream	*L. acidophilus, Bifidobacterium*	Regular and Low-Fat
Stonyfield Farms	Nonfat Frozen Yogurt	*L. bulgaricus, S. thermophilus, L. acidophilus, Bifidus, L. casei, L. reuteri*	After Dark Chocolate, Gotta Have Vanilla, Javalanche, Vanilla Fudge Swirl

Plain: 110 calories, 2.5 g fat, 1.5 g saturated fat, 10 mg cholesterol, 125 mg sodium, 12 g carbohydrate, 3 g fiber, 8 g sugar, 14 g protein, 300 mg calcium
Peach: 160 calories, 2 g fat, 1.5 g saturated fat, 10 mg cholesterol, 125 mg sodium, 25 g carbohydrate, 3 g fiber, 21 g sugar, 14 g protein, 300 mg calcium
Raspberry: 160 calories, 2 g fat, 1.5 g saturated fat, 10 mg cholesterol, 125 mg sodium, 25 g carbohydrate, 3 g fiber, 21 g sugar, 14 g protein, 300 mg calcium
Strawberry: 160 calories, 2 g fat, 1.5 g saturated fat, 10 mg cholesterol, 125 mg sodium, 25 g carbohydrate, 3 g fiber, 21 g sugar, 14 g protein, 300 mg calcium

Chocolate Crisp and Cool Mint Chocolate: 100 calories, 6 g fat, 4 g saturated fat, 0 mg cholesterol, 20 mg sodium, 11 g carbohydrate, 1 g fiber, 8 g sugar, 2 g protein, 200 mg calcium
Blueberry Vanilla: 100 calories, 6 g fat, 3.5 g saturated fat, <5 mg cholesterol, 25 mg sodium, 11 g carbohydrate, 1 g fiber, 9 g sugar, 2 g protein, 250 mg calcium
Yogurt and Granola Strawberry Bliss, Wild Berry, and Lemon Crème: 180 calories, 7 g fat, 3 g saturated fat, 0 mg cholesterol, 60 mg sodium, 24 g carbohydrate, 2 g fiber, 12 g sugar, 5 g protein, 200 mg calcium

170 calories, 2.5 g fat, 1 g saturated fat, 0 mg cholesterol, 100 mg sodium, 43 g carbohydrate, 12 g fiber, 10 g sugar, 4 g protein, 200 mg calcium

Regular: 120 calories, 5 g fat, 3 g saturated fat, 20 mg cholesterol, 390 mg sodium, 4 g carbohydrate, 4 g fiber, 3 g sugar, 13 g protein, 150 mg calcium
Low-Fat: 100 calories, 2.5 g fat, 1.5 g saturated fat, 15 mg cholesterol, 390 mg sodium, 4 g carbohydrate, 0 g fiber, 3 g sugar, 13 g protein, 150 mg calcium

Strawberry Banana Splash: 120 calories, 0 g fat, 0 g saturated fat, 0 mg cholesterol, 75 mg sodium, 25 g carbohydrate, 1 g fiber, 24 g sugar, 4 g protein, 150 mg calcium
Wild Berry Blast: 120 calories, 0 g fat, 0 g saturated fat, 0 mg cholesterol, 80 mg sodium, 25 g carbohydrate, 1 g fiber, 23 g sugar, 4 g protein, 150 mg calcium
Tropical Punch: 120 calories, 0 g fat, 0 g saturated fat, 0 mg cholesterol, 75 mg sodium, 25 g carbohydrate, 1 g fiber, 23 g sugar, 4 g protein, 150 mg calcium

Regular: 60 calories, 5 g fat, 3.5 g saturated fat, 20 mg cholesterol, 15 mg sodium, 1 g carbohydrate, 0 g fiber, 1 g sugar, 1 g protein, 40 mg calcium
Low-Fat: 35 calories, 2 g fat, 1 g saturated fat, 10 mg cholesterol, 25 mg sodium, 3 g carbohydrate, 0 g fiber, 2 g sugar, 1 g protein, 60 mg calcium

After Dark Chocolate: 100 calories, 0 g fat, 0 g saturated fat, <5 mg cholesterol, 60 mg sodium, 20 g carbohydrate, 0 g fiber, 18 g sugar, 4 g protein, 150 mg calcium
Gotta Have Vanilla: 100 calories, 0 g fat, 0 g saturated fat, <5 mg cholesterol, 70 mg sodium, 21 g carbohydrate, 0 g fiber, 19 g sugar, 4 g protein, 150 mg calcium
Javalanche: 100 calories, 0 g fat, 0 g saturated fat, <5 mg cholesterol, 65 mg sodium, 21 g carbohydrate, 0 g fiber, 18 g sugar, 4 g protein, 150 mg calcium
Vanilla Fudge Swirl: 120 calories, 0 g fat, 0 g saturated fat, <5 mg cholesterol, 65 mg sodium, 25 g carbohydrate, 0 g fiber, 22 g sugar, 4 g protein, 150 mg calcium

A Sample of Probiotic- and Prebiotic-Enhanced Foods Available in the United States—cont'd

Manufacturer	Product Name	Type of Probiotic/Prebiotic	Flavors
Stonyfield Farms	Low-Fat Frozen Yogurt	*L. acidophilus, Bifidus, L. casei, L. reuteri*	Cookies N' Dream, Crème Caramel, Minty Chocolate Chip, Raspberry White Chocolate Chunk
TCBY	Hand-Scooped Frozen Yogurt	*Lactobacillus acidophilus, Streptococcus thermophilus, Bifidobacterium lactis, Lactobacillus bulgaricus, Lactobacillus lactis, Lactobacillus paracasei, Lactobacillus rhamnosis*	Vanilla Bean, Chocolate Chunk Cookie Dough, Mint Chocolate Chunk, Chocolate Chocolate, Pralines and Cream, Strawberries and Cream, Butter Pecan, and Cookies and Cream
General Mills	Yo-Plus Yogurt	This product contains Optibalance which is the name for the unique *combination* of a prebiotic (3 grams of chicory root extract (inulin)) and probiotic (*Bifidobacterium lactis* Bb-12). The product also contains the live and active cultures *S.thermophilus* and *L. bulgaricus*	Strawberry, Cherry, Vanilla, Peach

Four Questions

Not all yogurts made in the United States currently list amounts of live and active cultures, but you can try to find out how much of the culture is in any product by contacting the manufacturer and asking these four important questions:

1. What health benefits have been documented for your product? Ask for specific reference citations or copies of articles that have been published. See if they are general review articles, or if they pertain to the specific strains of bacteria used in the product. General review articles are interesting but not relevant to the specific formulation being sold.

Nutrition Facts

Cookies N' Dream: 130 calories, 1 g fat, 0 g saturated fat, <5 mg cholesterol, 60 mg sodium, 25 g carbohydrate, 0 g fiber, 19 g sugar, 4 g protein, 150 mg calcium

Crème Caramel: 130 calories, 1.5 g fat, 1 g saturated fat, <5 mg cholesterol, 95 mg sodium, 26 g carbohydrate, 0 g fiber, 25 g sugar, 4 g protein, 150 mg calcium

Minty Chocolate Chip: 140 calories, 3 g fat, 1.5 g saturated fat, <5 mg cholesterol, 55 mg sodium, 24 g carbohydrate, 0 g fiber, 21 g sugar, 4 g protein, 150 mg calcium

Raspberry White Chocolate Chunk: 120 calories, 1.5 g fat, 1 g saturated fat, 0 mg cholesterol, 70 mg sodium, 22 g carbohydrate, 0 g fiber, 20 g sugar, 4 g protein, 150 mg calcium

Vanilla Bean: 120 calories, 3.5 g fat, 2 g saturated fat, 15 mg cholesterol, 60 mg sodium, 19 g carbohydrate, 0 g fiber, 16 g sugar, 3 g protein, 60 mg calcium

Chocolate Chunk Cookie Dough: 160 calories, 6 g fat, 3 g saturated fat, 15 mg cholesterol, 75 mg sodium, 24 g carbohydrate, 0 g fiber, 18 g sugar, 3 g protein, 100 mg calcium

Mint Chocolate Chunk: 140 calories, 5 g fat, 4 g saturated fat, 10 mg cholesterol, 55 mg sodium, 22 g carbohydrate, 0 g fiber, 18 g sugar, 3 g protein, 100 mg calcium

Chocolate Chocolate: 120 calories, 3.5 g fat, 2 g saturated fat, 15 mg cholesterol, 50 mg sodium, 14 g carbohydrate, <1 g fiber, 16 g sugar, 4 g protein, 100 mg calcium

Pralines and Cream: 140 calories, 4.5 g fat, 2 g saturated fat, 10 mg cholesterol, 80 mg sodium, 23 g carbohydrate, 0 g fiber, 19 g sugar, 3 g protein, 100 mg calcium

Strawberries and Cream: 120 calories, 2.5 g fat, 1.5 g saturated fat, 10 mg cholesterol, 50 mg sodium, 21 g carbohydrate, 0 g fiber, 18 g sugar, 2 g protein, 80 mg calcium

Butter Pecan: 110 calories, 4.5 g fat, 1.5 g saturated fat, 10 mg cholesterol, 90 mg sodium, 14 g carbohydrate, less than 1 g fiber, 11 g sugar, 4 g protein, 100 mg calcium

Cookies and Cream: 140 calories, 4 g fat, 2.5 g saturated fat, 10 mg cholesterol, 75 mg sodium, 22 g carbohydrate, 0 g fiber, 17 g sugar, 3 g protein, 100 mg calcium

110 calories, 1.5 g fat, 1 g saturated fat, 10 mg cholesterol, 70 mg sodium, 21 g carbohydrate, 3 g fiber, 16 g sugar, 4 g protein, 150 mg calcium

2. What levels of all probiotics contained in the product are present at the end of the shelf-life (assuming appropriate storage conditions)? Is this level the same as what was tested in human studies and shown to have a health benefit?

3. Does the company regularly survey its product to know that it meets the label claims once it is on the shelf?

4. Does the company use an objective, independent laboratory to certify that its product meets the label claims?

Reprinted with permission from U.S. Probiotics at www.usprobiotics.org.

Safe Handling?

There's one more unknown. Improper storage can kill probiotic bacteria, and you generally won't know how a product was handled prior to purchase. This shouldn't stop you from consuming prebiotic and probiotic foods. The same principle applies to many other foods we eat. Fruits and vegetables are exposed to heat, light, and air, and they lose a bit of nutritional value as time goes on. The bioavailability of calcium in a calcium-fortified beverage, for example, may be much less than what is reported on the label. Perhaps the beverage needs to be shaken for a minute to disperse the calcium before you drink it. If the food is otherwise healthful, go ahead and have it.

Bear in mind that you'll need to account for processing methods by asking questions of the manufacturer before selecting the right probiotic product for you. But even without a mechanism to establish the live probiotic

A Sample of Probiotic Products Sold Internationally

Manufacturer	Country	Product	Web Address
Yili	China	Yogurt	www.yili.com
Mengniu	China	Yogurt	www.mengniuir.com
Bright Dairy and Food	China	Yogurt, ice cream	www.brightdairy.com/e_main/index.php
Danone	France	Yogurt	www.danone.com
ProViva	Scandanavia	Fruit drink and yogurt	www.proviva.com
Meiji	Japan	Hard candies, cheesecake	www.meiji.com
Snow Brand Milk	Japan	Milk	www.snowbrand.co.jp
Valio Dairy	Finland	Yogurt	www.valio.fi/portal/page/portal/valiocom
Morinaga Milk Industry	Japan	Milk	www.morinagamilk.co.jp/menu/english.html
Fonterra	New Zealand	Yogurt	www.fonterra.com/wps/wcm/connect/fonterracom/fonterra.com/Home/
Yakult	Japan, UK, Argentina, Uruguay, some EU Nations	Dairy-based beverage	www.yakult.co.uk/Public/default.aspx

level at the time you consume the food, the probiotic foods recommended in this book are healthful in many other ways, since they are low-fat sources of protein and many are rich in calcium, potassium, zinc, and phosphorus.

International Appeal

The growing interest globally in functional foods is a strong testament to the link between diet and health. Probiotics have been well accepted in many countries for many years, with Japan accounting for over half of all functional food sales. To make an informed choice, you can and should ask the same four questions about any probiotic product available anywhere.

Established Health Benefits

The study of prebiotic and probiotic foods is a keen area of interest among digestive health researchers, so you're likely to find ongoing and in-progress studies on the very bacterium you are interested in. For years, researchers have known that immunity and disease have roots in the digestive tract. A meeting of the minds in 2006, attended by researchers from the Centers for Disease Control and Prevention, The National Institutes of Health, The Department of Health and Human Services, and many others, yielded these conclusions:

- Probiotics are living microorganisms that, upon ingestion, exert health benefits to their host.

- To be considered a probiotic, a microorganism must be viable and non-pathogenic, resistant to digestion, and associated with a health benefit.
- Prebiotics are non-digestible food ingredients that beneficially affect their host since they are available for fermentation in the colon.
- Prebiotics selectively stimulate the growth of "good" bacteria in the colon.
- There is strong evidence that both prebiotics and probiotics may help to reverse some of the effects of hypercholesterolemia.
- Probiotics have been linked with improving aspects of diarrheal diseases and lactose intolerance in humans.

The Unknowns
- What is the dosage needed to benefit health?
- How long are bacteria viable?

How Healthy Are They, Really?

Probiotic and prebiotic supplemented foods can be nutritious choices, especially for much-needed calcium. Yogurt, cottage cheese, and kefir provide lean protein and calcium, and most provide vitamin D as well to aid with calcium absorption. Calcium-rich foods are hard to come by in our diet. Although calcium is available in leafy greens and many fortified foods including soy milk, orange juice, and breakfast cereals, this is one mineral that we routinely run dangerously short on. Most people don't get enough calcium, a mineral important for bone density and the management of blood pressure. Adults age 31 to 50 should consume 1,000 mg of calcium per day; those who are 51 and older should consume 1,200 mg daily. The recipes in this book will ramp up your calcium intake with low-fat dairy, calcium-fortified tofu, and leafy greens.

Probiotic-enriched yogurt and some other products do have added sugar to improve flavor. But this is an instance where added sugar is beneficial to the food. Sweet taste is one of our strongest flavor preferences. When sugar is added to nutritious food, like a calcium-rich yogurt, to improve palatability, it is the ideal use of a sweetener! Is it too much sugar to allow the full benefit of the probiotic bacteria? Remember that it's what you eat over the course of the whole meal that will impact whether or not the bacteria survive. For example, if you were to drink 24 ounces of regular soda with your meal, the probiotic bacteria may not survive in your colon. We know that too much added sugar can feed bad bacteria, causing them to multiply and overtake the good bacteria in your colon. But the added sugar in yogurt is just the right amount to influence you to eat it regularly and not too much to affect the viability of beneficial probiotic bacteria. For more information on sugars and how much sugar you should be eating, see pp 61–62, "Too Much Sugar."

Survival of the Fittest Bacteria

Digestive acids in the stomach and small intestine can hamper the survival of probiotic bacteria before they reach the colon.

A high-sugar, high-fat, and high-meat diet can make it impossible for probiotic bacteria to survive. But studies also show that certain strains of probiotic bacteria don't survive processing well. A study published in *Immunology and Cell Biology* in 2000 looked at the survival of *L. acidophilus* and *Bifidobacterium*. The study found insufficient viability and survival of these bacteria in commercial food products and recommended further examination of processing methods to improve survival. This demonstrates the differences among bacterial species, the intrinsic characteristics of bacterial strains, and how some strains can ultimately survive processing, while some can't. The four questions that you ask the manufacturer about your food will help you decide whether or not you can rely on the manufacturing methods they use.

A 2001 study in the *American Journal of Clinical Nutrition* examined quality assurance criteria for probiotics. This study used the ability of the bacteria to stick to intestinal cells as a method for characterizing the strains and assessing the viability of bacteria in the intestinal tract. The probiotic bacterium must be able to adhere to the intestinal mucosa because this connection is necessary for bacterial colonization. This adhesion property can be unintentionally modified during processing of a probiotic-supplemented food and may be one of the quality control measures that your manufacturer uses to survey its product to verify that it meets the label claims.

How to Read a Study

You've located a research paper on the benefits of a particular probiotic bacterium for health; now what do you do? First, trust yourself to make sense of it. People without a medical background should still be able to draw conclusions from a scientific study. You can skip over the abstract; it's like a television commercial or advertisement for the study. It may not tell the full story and probably will include a bit of the researchers' opinions. They are entitled to them, but it's better to start elsewhere. Instead, skim the paper for an overview of key points and headings. This will frame the methods used and the thoroughness of the study. Now, scan the study from beginning to end and underline every word you don't know or understand. It might seem like overkill, but look up the words you don't understand. A simple Internet search will bring up a medical dictionary to shed light on unfamiliar terms. A good choice is the U.S. National Library of Medicine and the National Institutes of Health online medical dictionary at www.nlm.nih.gov/medlineplus/mplusdictionary.html. Be sure to note the context in which the words are used, since that can vary the meaning. Then, read the introduction and determine the purpose of the paper: the main objective or research question being posed. With this in mind, go back and read the paper, section by section, for comprehension. Take your time! When you get to the following sections, use this guide:

Methods: Try to get a picture in your mind of what was done at each step. Answer the question, what was actually measured?

Results: Look at the charts, figures, and tables, and try to translate them into plain English. It's easier than you think!

Discussion: These are the researcher's conclusions after completing the study. This section involves a lot of interpretation as the author reflects on the work and its meaning and how it relates to the field in general and to similar findings in other studies.

Reflection and Criticism: Here's where you become the research study critic and decide if the results mean anything to you! After summarizing the article, understanding the terms used, go back to the original research question and see if the methods and results bring you to the same conclusion.

The methods used, sample size, control groups, and many other factors in a study will help you decide whether or not it proves or disproves the study question. Here is a slightly more in-depth look at the various points of the article to use as a checklist as you analyze the research.

Purpose
1. What is the objective of the study?
2. What is the research question being posed?

The Four Questions... Answered

We've asked a sample of manufacturers to answer the four questions for many of these foods. Here's what we found:

Manufacturer	Product	What health benefits have been documented for your specific probiotic product?
Lifeway	Original Kefir, Low-fat Kefir, Nonfat Kefir	Kefir has been shown to improve lactose digestion and tolerance in adults with lactose maldigestion.
Lifeway	Organic Whole Milk, Organic Low-fat Milk	Stimulates protein digestion and appetite, decreases cholesterol content in blood, and improves salivation and excretion of stomach and pancreatic enzymes and peristalsis. It stimulates microphage production and improves immunity. Most favorable milk for people suffering from genetically stipulated lactose intolerance.
Attune	Wellness Bars	Help rebalance the digestive system, support a strong immune system, and improve overall feelings of well-being.
Kashi	Vive Cereal	Variety of digestive and overall health benefits. The same strain of probiotic that is in Kashi Vive has been studied in people with an intestinal disorder called symptomatic uncomplicated diverticular disease. Imbalances in intestinal microflora are thought to be related to the abdominal bloating and pain that frequently occurs with this disease. A recent study has shown that people who ate the probiotic strain in Kashi Vive had less intestinal discomfort than those who did not.
Stonyfield Farms	Frozen Yogurt	Enhance digestion, improve nutrient absorption, and enhance the body's defenses.

What levels of all probiotics contained in the product are present at the end of the shelflife (assuming appropriate storage conditions)? Is this level the same as what was tested in human studies and shown to have a health benefit?	Does the company regularly survey its product to know that it meets the label claims once it is on the shelf?	Does the company use an objective, independent laboratory to certify that its product meets label claims?
Five to 10 billion probiotics per one-cup serving until the end of shelflife. There is a bell curve in the value of bacteria available throughout the life of the product, which drops off dramatically at the end of shelflife.	Yes, the product is regularly surveyed.	Yes, an independent lab monitors production to ensure label claims are correct.
Five to 10 billion probiotics per serving until the end of shelflife. There is a bell curve in the value of bacteria available throughout the life of the product, which drops off dramatically at the end of shelflife.	Yes, the product is regularly surveyed.	Yes, an independent lab monitors production to ensure label claims are correct.
1010cfu/bar until the end of room temperature shelf-life.	Yes	Yes, a third-party lab is used to test company claims.
Approximately 1 billion probiotics per serving are present at the time of manufacture. The probiotics in Kashi Vive are stable when the cereal is stored in conditions typical to a home. In addition, as for all cereals, folding the inner liner of the carton when storing the cereal will help to keep it fresh.	Yes, we regularly test Kashi Vive to ensure we are meeting our stated claims.	Yes, a third-party laboratory is used to confirm that Kashi maintains nutritional value claims.
Our products meet or exceed the National Yogurt Association stipulations of at least 10 million cultures per gram at the time of manufacture. In addition, we have a longer shelf life: a 50- to 75-day shelf life without the use of preservatives. If stored at proper temperatures, we guarantee at least a 30-day shelf life with live active cultures intact.	Our product is tested throughout the production process, and in our warehouse, as it awaits shipment.	As certified organic products (and certified kosher by the Orthodox Union), we undergo rigorous inspections and certification by independent, outside agents. This certification includes random testing of ingredients and final products and on-site inspections.

The Four Questions. . . Answered—cont'd

Manufacturer	Product	What health benefits have been documented for your specific probiotic product?
TCBY	Frozen Yogurt	Strengthens the immune system, improves digestion, and stimulates better absorption of nutrients.
General Mills	Yo-Plus Yogurt	Yo-Plus contains a unique blend of the probiotic *Bifidobacterium lactis* Bb-12 and the prebiotic fiber inulin (chicory root extract). Together, they can help regulate digestive health. Bb-12 is one of the most widely studied probiotics. Over 55 human studies have been completed on Bb-12. Bb-12 has been shown to influence gastrointestinal health in a number of significant ways including improvements in diarrhea. Research has shown that 5 grams of inulin each day can help to maintain a healthy digestive system as part of a healthy diet and lifestyle.

What levels of all probiotics contained in the product are present at the end of the shelflife (assuming appropriate storage conditions)? Is this level the same as what was tested in human studies and shown to have a health benefit?	Does the company regularly survey its product to know that it meets the label claims once it is on the shelf?	Does the company use an objective, independent laboratory to certify that its product meets label claims?
The target is in excess of 10 million organisms per gram at production so that at the end of shelf-life we deliver a minimum of 1 million live active cultures per gram.	Yes, we have a strict quality control program in place, and we continuously review our products to ensure that any claims are capable of being substantiated.	Yes, part of our quality control program includes outside labs and suppliers for testing all of our products. We do periodic audits on each of our suppliers to make sure that they are following our protocols and continually compare to past audits to ensure they always maintain the high standards we hold for our company and products.
One serving of Yo-Plus provides at least 1 billion Bb-12 and 3 grams of inulin. Yo-Plus also provides the same amount of *S. thermophilus* and *L. bulgaricus* as other Yoplait yogurts.	Yes, we conduct routine analytical testing to confirm that our products are in compliance with U.S. Food and Drug Administration (FDA) labeling regulations.	Yes, we use certified methods to measure the number of live and active cultures in Yoplait products. In addition, we follow the National Yogurt Association (NYA) protocol to validate and register the results as required by the NYA to use the Live and Active culture seal. General Mills exceeds the criteria set by the NYA for the number of live and active cultures at time of manufacture and end of shelflife. General Mills uses internal standards and vendor-recommended testing to substantiate product content claims related to Bb-12. Our internal minimum requirement for Bb-12 is a billion per serving.

Design of the Study

1. What type of study was performed?
2. How was the study population sampled?
3. If it was a clinical trial, did they use a control group and did they randomize the results?

Measurement and Observation

1. Are there definitions of the terms used? There should be a list of the study's key words and definitions.
2. What are the outcome criteria?
3. What measurements were taken and how were they taken?
4. What method of validity or reliability was used?

Results

1. How are the data presented?
2. Are the data relevant to the study question?
3. Are there missing data that were not presented?

Conclusions

1. What are the main conclusions?
2. Is the study significant?
3. Is the study relevant to other populations?
4. Do any questions remain unsolved?

Once you've done your homework and decided on a specific product, pay attention to how it works for you. Keep in mind that we all have a unique physiology, a different composition of native intestinal flora, and distinctive nutritional status. We each might respond differently to different formulations.

If a product works for you, stick with it. If, after one month, a product does not work for you, try something else.

Probiotic Supplements and Procedures

Oh, if only a pill could lead the way to perfect health! After reading about the amazing health benefits of prebiotics and probiotics, you might be influenced to choose supplements. Maybe you'd like to eat whatever you want, even if it's not a diet that positively influences your digestive bacterial balance. If you hate eating fruits and vegetables but love high-fat foods and lots of meat, can you achieve the same bacterial balance with prebiotic or probiotic supplements and realize similar health benefits? Unfortunately, no.

Let's first look at the big picture of supplement use. The lure of a pill to cure every ill is too much for most people to pass up. It's easy to see why Americans spend billions of dollars every year on supplements. The claims on some supplement labels can be very enticing, and many of us open our wallet for pills with too-good-to-be-true claims such as these: "Stress Relief Formula," "Lose Weight Now," or "Joint Health Formula." It's tempting to throw caution to the wind and rely on a pill to make everything better, fight every disease, and cure every ache and pain.

Not so fast. It's well established that your digestive health is dependent on the foods you eat and the beverages you drink. Foods high in fat—particularly saturated, trans, and omega-6 fats—not only exclude healthful fiber-rich foods that feed your probiotic bacteria, but the good bacteria can't perform their functions adequately when overwhelmed with too much dietary fat. A diet high in meat can increase the level of amino compounds in your digestive tract, including nitrosamines, which influence enzyme patterns and upset the balance of bacteria in the colon. Too much added sugar is a problem as well. A diet rich in added sugar is often low in dietary fiber, and the added sugar can feed bad bacteria, allowing them to flourish over the good bacteria in your colon. What you eat is important to keep good bacteria alive and well, but it's a gamble to rely on probiotic supplements to set your balance straight. Quite simply, not enough is known about dosage or duration of use to safely recommend certain types of bacteria in the form of pills or powders for certain conditions.

According to the National Center for Complementary and Alternative Medicine at the National Institutes of Health, some probiotics have a long history of use without causing illness in people. However, they warn that probiotic supplement safety has not been thoroughly studied and that people with compromised immune systems, young children, and the elderly should proceed with caution.

Some of the side effects of probiotic supplements include gas, bloating, and sometimes more serious complications. They might cause infections that require treatment with antibiotics, particularly in people with underlying medical conditions. These supplements could actually cause too much stimulation of the immune system and even unintended gene transfer, the insertion of genetic material into a cell. Since the supplements are manufactured and regulated as foods, the U.S. Food and Drug Administration has special labeling requirements for them. Here are some important considerations:

- If you are thinking about using a probiotic product for an illness or condition for which you are under a physician's care, always ask permission from your physician first. No therapy should be used in place of conventional medical care, nor should you delay in seeking medical care when needed and rely on probiotic supplements instead.
- There are different strains of probiotics, and what holds true for one probiotic doesn't necessarily hold true for another, even when using a different preparation of the same strain of probiotic.
- If you have any side effects while using a probiotic product, seek attention from your physician.

Too Much of a Good Thing

It is possible to get too much of a good thing, even in a clinical setting. In a 2006 review published in the *American Journal of Clinical Nutrition*, the clinical use of probiotic supplements was examined. Probiotic bacteremia (the presence of bacteria in the bloodstream) occurred in patients with underlying immune compromise, chronic disease, or debilitation. In other words, these people were chronically sick and were likely trying to turn things around with probiotic supplements. But bacteremia is a pretty serious condition. It can present as a simple fever, but left untreated, it can lead to sepsis and septic shock, which requires aggressive treatment and has a pretty grim prognosis for recovery. Thankfully, most of these cases were resolved with antimicrobial therapy. All of these instances of probiotic bacteremia were in patients with preexisting intestinal pathology, meaning they were already suffering from chronic diarrhea or had had a surgical procedure on the intestines. Probiotics are recommended without much reservation as a treatment for diarrhea and for people who may have had surgery on their intestinal tract.

It's highly unlikely that you'll get too much probiotic bacteria by eating enhanced foods. But in many of the cases reported in this review, the probiotics were administered via a central venous line, bypassing the normal digestive process, which whittles down the presence of live bacteria before they reach the colon. The central line increased the likelihood of bacteremia by ferrying the bacteria to their destination without the benefit of digestion along the way. Here is a list of all the risk factors for probiotic bacteremia or sepsis. If you have one major factor and more than one of the minor factors, caution is recommended in using probiotic supplements:

Major Factors:
- Immune compromise, including a debilitated state or malignancy
- Premature infants

Minor Factors:
- Central venous line. This means that you are under a doctor's care and are receiving nourishment or medication through a central catheter line
- Impaired intestinal epithelial barrier (e.g., diarrheal illness or intestinal inflammation)
- Administration of probiotic directly into the small intestine
- Concomitant administration of broad-spectrum antibiotics to which probiotic is resistant (this means that antibiotics are administered at the same time to control population of the good bacteria, but the good bacteria are resistant to these antibiotics)
- Probiotics with properties of high mucosal adhesion or known pathogenicity
- Cardiac valvular disease (research shows that this applies only if you're taking the *Lactobacillus* strain of probiotics)

Colonic Infusion of Probiotic Bacteria

As you have learned, to reap the benefits of probiotic foods, the bacteria need to survive the stomach and small intestine to ferment in the colon. Is it possible to bypass this process and infuse bacteria directly into the colon? In 2003, a very small study of six patients with ulcerative colitis was published in the *Journal of Clinical Gastroenterology* and found that colonic intusion of probiotic bacteria proved helpful for all patients within four months of treatment. The results were positive for the six patients, and although the research is skimpy on the benefits for the larger group of people suffering from ulcerative colitis, it's an interesting area of research to watch.

Is Your Colon Really That Dirty?

Be aware, though, of the difference between this medical procedure— colonic infusion of probiotic bacteria, performed in a clinical setting—and at-home colonic "enhancements." A search on colon cleansing brings up well over a million hits, and photos and images that would make a nice addition to a horror movie. The Mayo Clinic recommendation is simple: Colon cleanses are unnecessary and could be harmful. So much is happening in our colon with regard to bacterial balance that it's hard to believe that anyone would want to disturb nature's way! But they do, and here's why it's not recommended: Your colon works beautifully on its own; digestion is truly one of the most amazing medical marvels. Your colon absorbs water and minerals and sets your electrolyte balance right, which controls some pretty

important body functions, such as heart rate, fluid balance, and oxygen delivery. Sometimes a colon cleanse disrupts this delicate balance, and long-term use of colon cleansing procedures can lead to anemia, malnutrition, and even heart failure. As for some supplements and these at-home cleanses, the best guidance you can use is your own good sense. If it seems too good to be true, it probably is.

Instead, do what you know will help your health the most. There's ample scientific evidence that what you eat has a big impact on your health and well-being. The recipes in this book are low-fat, meatless, and rich in fruits and vegetables, which is optimal for both digestive health and providing a suitable environment for your probiotic bacteria. If you are interested in trying a probiotic- and/or prebiotic-supplemented food, first identify the symptoms or condition you're trying to help (see p 42, "Probiotic Products with Targeted Health Benefits") and use your detective skills to ask the manufacturer the four questions about the food you're considering taking. New products hit the shelves regularly. If you're trying to treat a specific health condition or disease, read the research. Quality manufacturing, honest and straightforward marketing, and continued scientific knowledge will ensure that, some day, probiotics on your grocery shelf will have reliable and identifiable levels of bacteria cultures.

CHAPTER THREE

Getting Relief for Specific Illnesses and Diseases

Probiotics were originally defined as "live microorganisms which, when administered in adequate amounts, confer a health benefit on the host" by an expert consultation at a meeting convened by the Food and Agriculture Organization of the United Nations/World Health Organization in October 2001. Since then, numerous studies have documented the benefits of eating prebiotic- and probiotic-rich foods, with the most well-established being for relief of intestinal symptoms. According to research, a probiotic diet can help many ailments discussed on the following pages.

The Research Speaks

Research has probed far enough to reveal the specific health benefits of particular strains of probiotic bacteria. The names of the bacteria are all in Latin, with the genus as the first name and the species as the second. The genus identifies a family group of bacteria that have closely related functions, so a *Lactobacillus* species differs in function from a *Streptococcus* species. Here are some of the well-researched species and the diseases or conditions that they are reported to help:

Lactobacillus species	Health-Promoting Properties for These Diseases or Conditions
L. salivarius	Increases nutrient bioavailability (your body's ability to use the nutrient)
L. rhamnosus	Improves production of lactase and provides relief from symptoms of lactose intolerance. Relieves symptoms of and promotes recovery from diarrhea and constipation. Suppresses appearance of tumors and detoxifies carcinogens. Treats food allergies. Reduces risk of colon or bladder cancer. Treats urinary tract infections.
L. reuteri	Enhances immune response
L. plantarum	Treats colitis
L. paracasei	Relieves symptoms of and promotes recovery from diarrhea and constipation
L. lactis	Stimulates gastrointestinal immunity
L. johnsonii	Improves production of lactase and provides relief from symptoms of lactose intolerance

Lactobacillus species	Health-Promoting Properties for These Diseases or Conditions
L. gasseri	Restrains pathogen growth and translocation (movement from one place to another). Improves urogenital health. Relieves symptoms of and promotes recovery from diarrhea and constipation. Increases nutrient bioavailability (your body's ability to use the nutrient).
L. fermentum	Prevents or treats the effects of atopic dermatitis
L. casei	Reduces appearance of tumors and detoxifies carcinogens
L. acidophilus	Treats urinary tract infections. Treats candidiasis. Treats rheumatoid arthritis. Suppresses appearance of tumors and detoxifies carcinogens. Lowers blood cholesterol, low-density lipoprotein (LDL), and triglycerides. Improves production of lactase and provides relief from symptoms of lactose intolerance.

Streptococcus species	Health-Promoting Properties for These Diseases or Conditions
S. thermophilus	Suppresses appearance of tumors and detoxifies carcinogens. Reduces risk of colon or bladder cancer. Improves urogenital health. Relieves symptoms of and promotes recovery from diarrhea and constipation.

Bifidobacterium species	Health-Promoting Properties for These Diseases or Conditions
B. bifidum	Enhances immune response. Suppresses appearance of tumors and detoxifies carcinogens. Treats rheumatoid arthritis. Lowers blood cholesterol, low-density lipoprotein (LDL), and triglycerides.
B. breve	Lowers blood cholesterol, low-density lipoprotein (LDL), and triglycerides. Reduces chance of pathogen infection.
B. longum	Reduces risk of colon or bladder cancer
B. lactis	Relieves symptoms of and promotes recovery from diarrhea and constipation

Commercial Cures

Given the research on the specific benefits of particular probiotic bacteria, it's easy to see why it's important to know what's in a particular probiotic-enriched food to determine whether it will improve your symptoms. The following chart shows a sampling of foods and the illnesses they may help cure.

Probiotic Products with Targeted Health Benefits

Indicated Condition	Product	Strain
Infant diarrhea	Culturelle (capsules), Danimals (drinkable yogurt), DanActive (dairy drink)	*L. rhamnosus* GG, *L. casei* DN114001 (commercial strain designation "DefensisÔ")
Inflammatory bowel conditions	VSL#3 (powder)	Blend of 80% *S. thermophilus*, 4 strains of *Lactobacillus*, and 3 strains of *Bifidobacterium*
Antibiotic-associated diarrhea	Florastor (capsules), Culturelle (capsules), Danimals (drinkable yogurt)	*Saccharomyces cerevisiae* (boulardii) Lyo, *L. rhamnosus* GG
Irritable bowel syndrome	Align (capsules)	*B. infantis* 35624, *L. plantarum* 299V
Regulating gut transit time	Activia (yogurt)	*B. animalis* DN-173 010 (also called *Bifidus regularis*)
Keeping healthy	Stonyfield Farms (yogurt), DanActive, Yakult (dairy drink)	*L. reuteri* SD2112, *L. casei* DN114001, *L. casei* Shirota
Allergy in infants	Culturelle (capsules), Danimals (drinkable yogurt)	*L. rhamnosus* GG
Lactose intolerance	All yogurts that are not heat-treated after fermentation will contain these bacteria	*L. bulgaricus* and/or *S. thermophilus*
Immune support	Good Start Natural Cultures (infant formula), Culturelle (capsules), Danimals (drinkable yogurt), Stonyfield Farms (yogurt), DanActive (fermented milk), Naked Juice Probiotic Juice Smoothie	*B. lactis* Bb12, *L. casei* DN114001, *L. rhamnosus* GG, *L. reuteri* SD2112, *B. lactis* HN019 (HOWARU™ or DR10), *L. casei* DN114001, *B. lactis* HN019 (HOWARU™ or DR10)
Adjunct therapy during treatment for vaginal infections	Fem-Dophilus	*L. rhamnosus* GR-1 and *L. reuteri* RC-14
C. difficile colonization or toxin production in feces	Florastor	*Saccharomyces cerevisiae* (boulardii) Lyo

Reprinted with permission from U.S. Probiotics at www.usprobiotics.org.

How Do You Spell Relief?

In time, following a prebiotic and probiotic diet can help to turn things around for your general health and well-being. Even if you're healthy, it's worthwhile to follow the well-established disease-preventive diet spelled out with these recipes. The following information can help you manage specific conditions or disease and find some relief from aggravating symptoms. These recommendations are meant to provide you with an overview of the most current treatments available. As with any medical advice, always discuss any change in treatment with your physician first.

Overall Immunity

Aside from the digestive system, your body has a remarkable series of organs, specialized cells, and a circulatory system that work together to clear infection from your body. The clear fluid that flows through this system is called lymph, and it contains white blood cells. The lymph fluid bathes all the cells in the body, and the lymphatic vessels collect and move the fluid back into the blood circulation. Your blood and lymph vessels serve as a vehicle for immune cells and foreign molecules, and your immune cells circulate around the lymphatic system, searching for foreign antigens, exiting, and returning to the bloodstream once again to start over on the quest for invaders. Your lymph nodes work to control and move the

lymph fluid along, and the spleen plays a part in this process, providing a fort where immune system cells confront invading bacteria. Your bone marrow, thymus, and even your appendix house pockets of lymphoid tissue (including the lymph nodes, spleen, tonsils, and adenoids), which are a part of the body's immune system that helps protect it from bacteria and other invaders. This incredible process keeps you healthy from nearly any infection that you come into contact with.

Our intestinal bacteria are important for keeping the immune system healthy. Maybe you get sick more often than anyone you know, picking up every cold and virus that comes along. You might benefit from probiotics for improving your overall immunity. Intestinal bacteria maintain health by providing energy, nutrients, and protection against invaders.

Probiotics play a role in managing the balance of bacteria to provide optimal immune protection. A 2007 study published in the *European Journal of Clinical Nutrition* found that *L. acidophilus* and *B. lactis* supplemented in yogurt survived digestion and increased phagocytic (cells that ingest and destroy foreign matter) activity to help tame harmful bacteria. A 2007 study published in the *Journal of Nutrition* showed positive natural killer (NK) cell activity—a marker for good health—in ten healthy volunteers taking a three-week daily dose of *L. casei* strain Shirota. An increasing number of experiments reveal the capacity of intestinal bacteria to interact with your immune system.

Diarrhea

Diarrhea can have many causes, including a bacterial or viral infection, serious illness such as AIDS, parasites, medications, and food intolerances. Many times, diarrhea clears up on its own after just a few loose stools. It's marked by cramps, bloating, nausea, and an urgent need to have a bowel movement. If diarrhea is accompanied by the following serious symptoms, seek medical care immediately: fever, severe pain in the abdomen or rectum, blood in the stool, severe diarrhea for more than three days, or symptoms of dehydration that include dry or sticky mouth, low or no urine output, concentrated urine that appears dark yellow, not producing tears, or sunken eyes.

Some food and drink can occasionally cause diarrhea. Consider eliminating any of these offending foods, drinks, and drugs to control your diarrhea:

Irritating Substances

Food, Drink, or Drug	Offending Ingredient
Apple juice, pear juice, sugar-free gum, sugar-free mints	Hexitols, sorbitol, mannitol
Apple juice, pear juice, grapes, honey, dates, nuts, figs, soft drinks (especially fruit flavors)	Fructose
Table sugar	Sucrose
Milk, ice cream, yogurt, frozen yogurt, soft cheese, chocolate	Lactose

Food, Drink, or Drug	Offending Ingredient
Antacids containing magnesium	Magnesium
Coffee, tea, cola, some headache medications	Caffeine
Light or nonfat potato chips, ice cream, or baked goods	Olestra

If you have diarrhea, be sure to drink plenty of fluids. Sometimes, bland foods such as rice, cereal, crackers, and bread are better tolerated and reduce episodes of diarrhea. There are also medications available over the counter to control diarrhea and help you feel better, including:

- **Loperamide** (one brand name is Imodium). Don't take this medication if you have bloody or black stools; seek medical attention instead.
- **Bismuth subsalicylate** (brand names: Kaopectate, Pepto-Bismol). Don't take this medication if you have an allergy to aspirin.

Sometimes people experience diarrhea for longer than three days, but they're unwilling to treat the diarrhea since they are encouraged that they may be losing weight. Diarrhea is not the way to lose weight. You won't lose stored fat this way, and with diarrhea lasting more than three days, you put yourself at risk for dehydration or electrolyte imbalance.

If you have chronic diarrhea, a specific food may be to blame. Keep a food log and try to pinpoint the offending food. Diarrhea can be a side effect of a sensitivity or intolerance to lactose, yeast, gluten, fructose, or other foods. When you seek medical treatment, bring your log with you.

The duration of diarrhea caused by gastroenteritis was shortened in studies using probiotics including *L. casei* GG, *L. reuteri,* and *S. boulardii*. A combination probiotic including *L. casei, L. bulgaricus*, and *S. thermophilus* can help alleviate antibiotic-induced diarrhea.

Constipation

Constipation is marked by three or fewer bowel movements per week. The stool can be hard and dry and is usually difficult to pass. Here are some ways to avoid constipation:

- Eat fruits, vegetables, and whole grains.
- Drink plenty of water and other liquids.
- Exercise regularly.
- Don't hurry! If you have an urge to have a bowel movement, get to the bathroom and take as much time as necessary once you're there.
- Use laxatives only on the advice of your physician.
- Rule out your medications as a cause for constipation.

It is not recommended that you take laxatives for constipation unless you're directed by a physician to take them. Overuse or long-term use of laxatives can damage the colon, decreasing the natural ability of your colon to contract and damaging nerves, muscles, and tissues of the colon, and this sometimes worsens constipation. If you have any change in bowel habits, or if you have constipation for more than seven days accompanied by rectal bleeding, seek medical attention.

There are dozens of promising studies about the effectiveness of probiotics for alleviating constipation. Studies show the probiotic *L. casei rhamnosus* is helpful in alleviating chronic constipation in children, and the probiotic *E. coli* strain Nissle 1917 is well tolerated and helps improve gastrointestinal complaints including constipation, inflammatory bowel disease, and irritable bowel syndrome. According to a 2006 study published in *Acta Biomed*, the probiotic *B. longum* regulates gastrointestinal transit time, increases intestinal water content, and improves constipation.

Lactose Intolerance

Lactose intolerance affects 80 percent of African-Americans, 80 to 100 percent of American Indians, and 90 to 100 percent of Asians. The symptoms include bloating, gas, abdominal pain, and even diarrhea. These symptoms are caused by the fermentation of lactose, a milk sugar, in the colon. The lactose sits undigested, since these people lack the enzyme, called lactase, required to break it down into glucose and galactose. *L. rhamnosus* or *L. johnsonii* can help to manage these symptoms. Here are a few other strategies to get better control over your lactose intolerance:

- Check product labels for hidden sources of lactose including whey, nonfat dry milk, curds, or dry milk solids. These ingredients are found in many foods, sometimes where you least expect to find them, such as cereal, lunch meats, and salad dressings.
- Use lactase enzyme tablets or drops to help break down the lactose. Follow package directions for dosage, and be sure to take them just before eating, or in the case of drops, with your first bite of food.
- Get enough calcium from other sources, such as sardines, leafy green vegetables including spinach or broccoli, pinto beans, salmon, or calcium-fortified orange juice. Many people with lactose intolerance can tolerate yogurt, which has plenty of calcium.
- Consider taking a supplement with calcium and vitamin D. If you're taking other medications, ask your physician first.

Ulcerative Colitis

Colitis symptoms vary from person to person. Although some people have months or years of remission from symptoms, many times symptoms return periodically or chronically. The goal of treatment is to provide relief from these symptoms, which can include fatigue, weight loss, loss of appetite, skin lesions, bloody diarrhea, nausea, and abdominal cramps. Unfortunately, the cause of ulcerative colitis is unknown. With permission from your physician, consider using the probiotic *L. plantarum* to alleviate symptoms. A study published in the *Journal of Gastroenterology and Hepatology* in 2006 reported improved immunomodulatory activity when using this probiotic, which may reduce inflammation in the colon. Current treatment includes drug therapy using primarily three forms of drugs:

- **Aminosalicylates.** Most people with mild-to-moderate symptoms are treated with this group of drugs first, and they are also used to treat a relapse. Sulfasalazine is effective, and if you experience side effects to this drug, the next options are olsalazine, mesalamine, and balsalazide.
- **Corticosteroids.** If the aminosalicylates are not effective, people with mild-to-moderate symptoms may be prescribed a short course of corticosteroids such as prednisone, methylprednisone, and hydrocortisone, which also reduce inflammation. These are prescribed for short-term use only since they may cause serious side effects in the long term, such as weight gain, acne, facial hair, hypertension, diabetes, mood swings, bone mass loss, and an increased risk of infection.
- **Immunomodulators.** These reduce inflammation by affecting the immune system, and they include azathioprine and 6-mercapto-purine. The drugs are slow acting, and it may take up to six months before symptoms improve.

Speak to your doctor about trying a new type of drug if you are dissatisfied with your current regimen. Surgery to remove the colon, also known as a proctocolectomy, is necessary in 25 to 40 percent of patients with ulcerative colitis. To prevent post-surgery complications, including a common infection of the ostomy known as pouchitis, studies are being conducted on VSL#3, a high-concentration probiotic preparation of eight live freeze-dried bacterial species that are normal components of the human gastrointestinal bacteria, including four strains of *Lactobacilli* (*L. casei, L. plantarum, L. acidophilus,* and *L. delbrueckii* sub-species bulgaricus), three strains of *Bifidobacteria* (*B. longum, B. breve,* and *B. infantis),* and *Streptococcus salivarius* sub-species thermophilus. A large, well-designed clinical trial is in order to see if these bacteria provide protection.

If you're facing surgery or treatment for ulcerative colitis, it's worthwhile to gather as much information as possible. Speak to your doctor, nurse, and others with the disease. For support, and to weigh your treatment options, visit the Crohn's and Colitis Foundation of America Web site at www.ccfa.org. You can participate in a live chat, phone in for help, and read up on the recent research and head-lines about your disease.

Crohn's Disease

Crohn's disease is a classic case of not knowing which came first. Is the reaction in the intestines of Crohn's sufferers to "attack" all invaders including bacteria, food, and other substances the *cause* of the disease, or does inflammation cause the disease to start in the first place? Even though the etiology of this disease is a mystery, the symptoms are no less aggravating. Those suffering from Crohn's usually experience abdominal pain and diarrhea, although they sometimes suffer from rectal bleeding, weight loss, fever, arthritis, or skin problems, too. Some people with Crohn's have long periods of remission, sometimes even years, and drug therapy is in order for many Crohn's sufferers. Here's a list of drugs that may help:

- **Anti-inflammation drugs.** The first line of treatment is usually a drug containing mesalamine that helps control inflammation. Mesalamine-containing drugs include Asacol, Dipentum, or Pentasa.
- **Cortisone or steroids.** Drugs such as prednisone are sometimes prescribed, particularly when the disease is first diagnosed. These drugs can have severe side effects, as noted above.
- **Immune system suppressors.** These drugs suppress the immune system, and they include 6-mercaptopurine or a related drug, azathioprine. They are sometimes used with steroids.
- **Infliximab (Remicade).** If you don't respond to standard treatment, this new group of medications may provide relief from symptoms of moderate-to-severe Crohn's disease.

- **Antibiotics.** These may be used to treat bacterial overgrowth in the small intestine caused by stricture, fistulas, or prior surgery. These drugs usually include ampicillin, sulfonamide, cephalosporin, tetracycline, or metronidazole.
- **Anti-diarrheal and fluid replacements.** Some of the anti-diarrheal drugs used include diphenoxylate, loperamide, and codeine. Those who lose too much fluid from diarrhea are treated with fluid and electrolyte replacement.

For as many as 75 percent of people suffering from Crohn's disease, surgery is eventually required when medication can no longer control symptoms. There are no foods that are known to cause Crohn's disease, but for some people, the following foods increase diarrhea and cramping: bulky grains, hot spices, alcohol, and milk products. Studies continue on probiotic use for relief of symptoms of Crohn's and all inflammatory bowel diseases.

Rheumatoid Arthritis

Treatment for rheumatoid arthritis (RA) varies according to the symptom, and the symptoms run the gamut. Some of these include fatigue, fever, stiffness, flu-like symptoms, muscle pain, loss of appetite, weight loss, and anemia. Studies show promise for the treatment of RA, with two probiotics, *B. bifidum* and *L. acidophilus*, leading the way.

It's important that you have the right health care team, including a rheumatologist—a physician specializing in diseases of the bone, muscle, and joints. Your team may also include an occupational therapist, a nurse, a physical therapist, and a psychologist. Here are the main categories of drugs that are sometimes used to treat RA:

- **Non-steroidal anti-inflammatory drugs (NSAIDs).**These include aspirin, ibuprofen, indomethacin, and COX-2 inhibitors such as valdecoxib and celecoxib, and they're used to reduce inflammation and control pain.
- **Analgesic drugs.** Drugs such as acetaminophen, propoxyphene, meperidine, and morphine are sometimes recommended to relieve pain.
- **Glucocorticoids or prednisone.** These are prescribed in low doses to reduce inflammation and slow joint damage.
- **Disease modifying antirheumatic drugs (DMARDs).** Together with NSAIDs and/or prednisone, these are prescribed to slow joint destruction caused by RA over time. These drugs include methotrexate, injectable gold, penicillamine, azathioprine, chloroquine, hydroxychloroquine, sulfasalazine, and oral gold. Recent studies have shown that the most aggressive treatment for controlling RA may be the combination of methotrexate and biologic response

modifiers. The dual drug combination seems to create a more effective treatment, especially for people who may not have success with—or who have built up a resistance to—methotrexate or another drug alone. Doctors now are prescribing combination drug therapy, such as this dual drug treatment, and it appears that these combination drug therapies might become the newest treatment protocol for RA.

- **Biologic response modifiers.** This class of drugs may be prescribed to modify the immune system by inhibiting cytokines, which are proteins that contribute to inflammation. Examples of these are etanercept, infliximab, adalimumab, and anakinra.

Some people with RA subscribe to protein-A immunoadsorption therapy, which filters your blood to remove antibodies and immune complexes that support inflammation. Surgical options for treating RA include:

- synovectomy, or removal of the diseased synovium, or joint lining
- arthroscopic surgery to repair and remove tissues, primarily in the knee and shoulder
- joint replacement or arthroplasty, which involves removal of the joint and replacement with a synthetic joint
- arthrodesis, in which two bones are fused together to provide stability in the spine, wrists, ankles, fingers, or toes

Candidiasis

This is a yeast infection you can get from a fungus that lives almost everywhere. Most of the time, your body keeps the fungus under control unless you're sick or taking antibiotics; then it can flourish and cause an infection of the skin, vagina, mouth, or (most seriously) bloodstream. A combination of probiotics shows some promise in controlling oral *Candida* and decreased salivation in the elderly, but studies are not as promising on the effectiveness of oral *L. acidophilus* for vulvovaginal *Candida* infections. To treat vaginal infections of this type, some women try home remedies including vinegar douches, tea tree oil cream, and vaginal suppositories made with garlic or boric acid. The Mayo Clinic warns that even though some women report relief from symptoms by using these remedies, well-designed, randomized, controlled trials are needed to determine both the safety and effectiveness of these therapies. Instead, Mayo doctors recommend conventional treatment including antifungal creams and suppositories. There is some encouraging research about the effectiveness of *L. acidophilus* suppositories as a treatment.

Urinary Tract Infections

Some of the symptoms of a urinary tract infection (UTI) include a frequent urge to use the bathroom and pain or burning when you go; fever, tiredness, or shakiness; urine that has an odor or is cloudy or reddish in color;

and pain the lower abdomen. The standard treatment is antibiotics. The probiotics *L. rhamnosus* and *L. acidophilus* hold promise for treating UTIs, but more research is needed to determine dosage guidance.

Cranberries have been tested as a preventive measure against UTI, but the studies were small, some were not randomized or controlled, and the results are not conclusive. The cranberry is thought to prevent bacteria, such as *E. coli*, from clinging to the cell walls along the urinary tract. The National Center for Complementary and Alternative Medicine at the National Institutes of Health warns that you shouldn't rely on cranberry juice to treat an infection, nor should you drink large quantities of cranberry juice because this can cause gastrointestinal upset or diarrhea. If you want to try drinking cranberry juice for prevention, limit your intake to just 8 ounces per day. This will help you to avoid squeezing out more nutritious foods in your day and to keep the amount of added sugar to a minimum.

High Cholesterol

According to the American Heart Association, the following tips are a good starting point to get blood cholesterol under control. (See chapter 4: Nutrition for Digestive Health, for more details about healthful fats and fiber to help control cholesterol.)

- Schedule a cholesterol screening.
- Eat foods low in saturated fat and trans fat.
- Choose omega-3 and unsaturated fats.
- Maintain a healthy weight.
- Exercise regularly.
- Follow your doctor's advice.

Your doctor may prescribe medication to lower your cholesterol or help raise your HDL (high-density lipoprotein) cholesterol, which can help to control your total cholesterol and LDL cholesterol levels. These may be prescribed individually or in combination with other drugs.

Various medications can lower blood cholesterol levels. They may be prescribed individually or in combination with other drugs.

- **Clofibrate (Atromid-S).** This drug raises the HDL ("good") cholesterol levels and lowers triglyceride levels.
- **Gemfibrozil (Lopid).** This drug raises HDL cholesterol levels.
- **Nicotinic acid.** This drug lowers triglycerides and LDL cholesterol and raises HDL cholesterol.*

  *Niacin (nicotinic acid). Use caution with niacin! Sometimes people try to purchase dietary supplements to perform the same function as prescription niacin, and this is dangerous! Dietary supplements vary according to dosage, and it's easy to get too much. Too much niacin, also known as vitamin B3, can cause itchiness, cramps, and nausea, and it can be toxic and cause liver failure. Always rely on your doctor's advice and use prescription-only versions of niacin.

- **Resins.** These drugs work in the intestines by binding to bile acids and helping to remove cholesterol. Three of these drugs are cholestyramine (Questran, Prevalite, Lo-Cholest), colestipol (Colestid), and colesevelam (WelChol).
- **Statins.** Statin drugs are commonly prescribed to lower LDL ("bad") cholesterol levels. They interrupt the formation of cholesterol from the circulating blood. The most commonly prescribed statins include atorvastatin (Lipitor), fluvastatin (Lescol), lovastatin (Mevacor), pravastatin (Pravachol), rosuvastatin calcium (Crestor), simvastatin (Zocor).

The probiotics *L. plantarum, S. thermophilus,* and *L. bulgaricus* show promise in modulating cholesterol levels. You can also focus on prebiotic soluble fiber–rich foods such as fruits, oatmeal, and beans, which you'll find well represented in these recipes, to lower blood cholesterol level with diet.

High Blood Pressure

According to the National Heart, Lung, and Blood Institute, a blood pressure reading of

- 120/80 or lower is normal blood pressure
- Between 120 and 139 for the top number, or systolic, or between 80 and 89 for the bottom number, or diastolic, is pre-hypertension
- 140/90 or higher is high blood pressure

High blood pressure is known as a silent killer since it usually doesn't have any symptoms, but some people do report chronic headaches with high blood pressure. It can cause serious problems such as stroke, heart attack, blindness, and kidney failure. The good news is that you can control high blood pressure with diet and lifestyle. Here are some strategies for getting your blood pressure under control:

- Don't smoke.
- Eat a diet rich in fruits, vegetables, and low-fat dairy, and control your sodium intake.
- Maintain a healthy weight. Sometimes losing only ten pounds, even if you have much more weight to lose, can significantly lower your blood pressure.
- Get 30 minutes of activity on most days of the week.
- Limit your alcohol intake to one drink a day for women or two drinks a day for men.

DASH, the Dietary Approach to Stop Hypertension, recommends that you start with a limit of 2,300 mg sodium per day, and if you still need to lower your blood pressure, limit sodium to 1,500 mg per day. Your prebiotic and probiotic recipes will help to control blood pressure since they are rich in low-fat dairy and fruits and vegetables.

According to the Mayo Clinic, if you have pre-hypertension, lifestyle factors are your first line of defense. It may sound like old-fashioned advice, but a diuretic (usually a thiazine)—which helps rid your body of excess fluid and, in turn, can lower your blood pressure and make it easier for your heart to pump—may be the first pill prescribed to help control hypertension. This is usually prescribed along with a recommendation to heed the healthy lifestyle advice as well. If this doesn't work, and you have blood pressure higher than 160/100, your doctor may recommend that you take one of the following medications in addition to the diuretic and lifestyle changes.

- **Beta blockers.** These work by reducing nerve signals to the heart and blood vessels, thus lowering blood pressure.
- **Angiotensin-converting enzyme (ACE) inhibitors.** These block the production of a hormone that causes blood vessels to narrow, thus helping blood vessels relax.
- **Angiotensin II receptor blockers.** These act on the hormone angiotensin, which works to constrict blood vessels. This medication allows blood vessels to widen instead.
- **Calcium channel blockers.** When calcium goes into heart and blood vessel muscle cells, it can raise blood pressure. This medication blocks this action, causing the cells to relax.

More studies are needed to confirm whether or not the probiotic *L. johnsonii* La1 is helpful to modulate blood pressure.

Colon Cancer

Colon cancer, also known as colorectal cancer or rectal cancer, is the fourth most common cancer in both men and women in the United States. The cause is still a mystery, but it can present as blood in the stool, narrower stools, a change in bowel habits, and general stomach discomfort. Treatment of this cancer usually involves radiotherapy, chemotherapy, and surgery, or some combination of these.

Probiotics including *L. rhamnosus, S. thermophilus*, and *B. longum* are being studied to prevent colon cancer. A 2006 study published in the *Journal of Nutrition* noted promise in the use of *B. longum* for reducing inflammation and the risk of colon cancer. In many of the studies, the benefit of using the probiotics for reducing colon cancer risk is enhanced by the use of prebiotic foods.

It's also a good idea to eat less meat, since a diet rich in meat is connected to higher incidence of colon cancer. A high-meat diet can cause an overload of amino compounds and nitrosamines in the digestive tract, which leads to changed enzyme patterns that alter colonic bacteria. All of these diet recommendations will be easy to accomplish with these prebiotic and probiotic recipes.

Atopic Dermatitis

"Atopic dermatitis" actually means a tendency to develop allergy conditions and swelling of the skin. The symptoms can include redness, swelling, cracking, weeping of clear fluid, crusting, thick skin, or scaling of the skin. Although the cause is not known, it can be genetic, and people suffering from this skin condition often live in cities or dry climates and also suffer from environmental allergies such as hay fever or have asthma. There are many environmental considerations when treating and trying to avoid symptoms of atopic dermatitis, including avoiding these common irritants:

- Skin contact with wool or man-made fibers
- Irritating soaps, perfumes, and makeup, chlorine and mineral oil
- Dust, sand, and cigarette smoke

Atopic dermatitis can also result from foods, plants, animals, or airborne allergens such as

- Eggs, fish, milk, peanuts, soy products, and wheat
- Dust mites
- Mold
- Pollen
- Dog or cat dander

Stress can aggravate atopic dermatitis, but it hasn't been shown to cause it. Skin infections, temperature, and climate can also lead to skin flare-ups. Here are some simple things that you can do to reduce flare-ups:

- Use a moisturizer after a bath or shower, and avoid long, hot baths or showers.
- Avoid a dry climate in the winter or a dry year-round climate.
- Avoid going from sweating to being chilled.
- Avoid bacterial infections.

Develop a good skin-care routine, follow it closely, and treat symptoms as soon as they occur. Some people take antihistamines at bedtime to avoid nighttime scratching. The medications that are sometimes prescribed include corticosteroids and antibiotics to treat bacterial infections.

Some people benefit from light therapy or a mixture of light therapy and a drug called psoralen. The studies relating to relief from atopic dermatitis from probiotic use are mixed but encouraging.

Bladder Cancer

Smoking is a major risk factor for bladder cancer (see chapter 5: Live Well for Digestive Health, for tips on how to stop smoking and reduce your risk). The risk for bladder cancer is higher in older white males and for those with a family history of bladder cancer. Here are some of the signs and symptoms:

- Blood in urine
- Frequent urge to urinate
- Pain when you urinate
- Lower-back pain

Treatment for bladder cancer includes surgery, chemotherapy, radiation, and immunotherapy, which is sometimes called biological therapy.

A 2007 report in *Der Urologe*, a German medical journal, noted a connection between permanent hair dyes and increased risk of bladder cancer. Hair dye can expose you to arylamine, a substance that must be detoxified by the skin and liver. Some studies show that people with a high fluid intake have a 50 percent decreased risk for bladder cancer. There is compelling research about the effectiveness of probiotics to reduce the risk for bladder cancer or to reduce the recurrence rate. The probiotic *L. casei* strain Shirota is particularly intriguing, and the probiotic *L. plantarum* is being studied for benefit against urogenital post-surgical infections.

While it's true that there is much we don't know about dosage for probiotics or the exact process by which they help disease or illness, there are currently hundreds of studies in progress on the subject of probiotics. Take matters into your own hands with lifestyle changes that can alleviate symptoms of any of these diseases or conditions. Prebiotic and probiotic foods are well-established health-promoting foods and are easy to include in your daily diet with the help of these recipes. A healthful diet like this one can help you manage a multitude of symptoms and prevent many diseases.

CHAPTER FOUR

Optimizing Nutrition for Digestive Health

Your probiotic and prebiotic diet is simply a sensible diet. It's similar to the diet recommended for prevention of cardiovascular disease and some cancers, for weight management, and for digestive health. This diet includes fiber-rich whole grains and plenty of vegetables and fruit, and it is meatless and low in sugar and fat. Soon you'll be enjoying the benefits of balanced digestive bacteria, including reduced risk for disease, improved immunity, and improved digestive health (meaning fewer bouts of diarrhea and constipation).

Fruit and Veggies: Serve 'Em Up

The United States Department of Agriculture (USDA) proclaims that fruits and vegetables are so important for digestive health, you should eat at least five servings a day. The good news is that one serving of produce is pretty tiny. For fruit, it's about 60 calories' worth, and for vegetables, about 20 calories. When you put the amounts in perspective, the servings of produce add up quickly!

It's easy to meet your minimum requirement for the best digestive health. The more calories you take in, the more produce you should eat. Here's a guide to help you be sure

SERVING STATS

One serving of fruit equals one medium-sized whole fruit, 1 cup (130 g) berries, ½ cup (75 g) grapes, 2 tablespoons (30 g) dried fruit, 2 plums, 1 kiwi, or ½ cup (120 ml) fruit juice.

One serving of vegetables equals 1 to 2 cups (20 to 40 g) leafy vegetables, 1 cup (135 g) non-leafy vegetables, ½ cup (80 g) cooked vegetables, or ¾ cup (175 ml) low-sodium tomato juice.

you're getting enough produce every day based on your calorie intake:

Calorie Level: 1,500
Fruit: 2 servings
Vegetables: 4 servings

Calorie Level: 1,000
Fruit: 2 servings
Vegetables: 4 servings

Calorie Level: 1,700
Fruit: 2 servings
Vegetables: 5 servings

Calorie Level: 1,800
Fruit: 2 servings
Vegetables: 5 servings

Calorie Level: 1,900
Fruit: 2 servings
Vegetables: 5 servings

Calorie Level: 2,000
Fruit: 2 servings
Vegetables: 5 servings

Fruits and vegetables are nutritional kings and queens. They provide fiber, which moves food through your digestive system, and help feed probiotic bacteria in your colon. A diet rich in fruits and vegetables is recommended for reducing your risk for many forms of cancer, heart disease, and other diseases, as well as for weight loss. Although the nutritional values of some fruits and vegetables trump others, there's no such thing as an unhealthy choice of produce. Even the vegetable with the lowest nutrient content will still provide fiber, water, and some phytochemicals to help fight disease. In these recipes, you'll find plenty of fruits and vegetables.

Tips on Choosing Organic Produce

Vegetables and fruits are at the crux of eating for optimal digestive health, but you may be confused about whether or not to choose organically grown produce. Your grocery store and health-food market have rows of tempting, delicious produce. For the best digestive health, it's worthwhile to choose organic produce or locally grown, conventionally farmed fresh produce.

Pesticide residue on produce can kill probiotic bacteria. If your probiotic bacteria are going to survive digestion, you'll need to remove as many barriers as possible along the way. Conventionally raised produce has higher amounts of pesticide residue than organic produce.

In fact, organic produce should be free of pesticide residue, but traces of pesticide residue can sometimes contaminate organic produce if pesticides drifted into the field and settled on the organic produce from a nearby conventional farming field or if the organic produce was stored with conventionally farmed produce. But this pesticide residue on organic produce is rare. The good news is that you can wash your conventionally grown local farm-fresh produce to remove some of the pesticide residue.

Rinse and Rub to Remove the Grub

Whether you buy conventionally farmed or organic produce, wash your hands and the produce before preparing to eat. Under cool running water, use your hands and a soft vegetable brush to lightly scrub the surface of the produce. Do this for all produce, including produce with a thick skin, such as cantaloupe, since cutting into the produce can introduce bad bacteria or pesticide residue inside on the edible portion. Spend at least ninety seconds rinsing and rubbing.

Organic produce usually has a little more nutritional value than conventionally grown produce. Studies show slightly higher levels of vitamin C in organic produce, for example. But the nutritional value of any fresh produce declines a little each day after it's picked. If you can get locally grown, farm-fresh produce, the nutritional value can be just as good as organic produce that takes five days or more in travel time to be delivered to your market.

Go Green

Organic produce is grown using environmentally friendly farming methods. By choosing organic, you'll also get a chance to try more unique produce, giving some variety and taste to your diet. If you're environmentally conscious, you'll want to consider all factors. For example, if the organic produce is grown across the country, you might want to consider the environmental impact of the fuel used and truck exhaust created to deliver it to you.

No matter which produce you choose, the important thing is that you're choosing fruits and vegetables, which provide an optimal environment in your digestive tract for prebiotic and probiotic activity and the best possible digestive health.

Nutrition Fact Finding

Fruits and vegetables don't usually come with nutrition facts labels attached. But with packaged foods, you'll have to do some label reading to find healthful ingredients for your prebiotic and probiotic recipes. When you're scanning your nutrition facts label, visit this website for tips on what to look for:

www.cfsan.fda.gov/~dms/foodlab.html

THE HIGHS AND LOWS OF PESTICIDE RESIDUE ON CONVENTIONAL PRODUCE

Highest in Pesticide Residue

Apples
Bell Peppers
Celery
Cherries
Imported Grapes
Nectarines
Peaches
Pears
Potatoes
Red Raspberries
Spinach
Squash
Strawberries

Lowest in Pesticide Residue

Asparagus
Avocado
Bananas
Broccoli
Cauliflower
Corn (sweet)
Kiwi
Mango
Onions
Papaya
Pineapple
Sweet Peas
Watermelon

Whole Grains

Food labels will help you select whole-grain foods. Whole grains are important for good digestive health. The prebiotic, fiber-rich foods you eat, like those found in these recipes, feed your probiotic bacteria, keeping them alive and active in your colon.

If you've tried any recent low-carbohydrate diet trends that drastically limit carbohydrates, it's unlikely that you're getting enough fiber and whole grains, a critical factor for probiotic viability in the colon. In a 2004 review of low-carbohydrate diets in the *Lancet*, the success of low-carbohydrate diets was attributed to the monotony and simplicity of the diet, which inhibits choices and food intake. Also, protein has a satiating effect and can decrease overall calorie intake. Although it's tempting to try these quick-fix diets to drop pounds, it's what you eat over the course of years that really counts, so stay away from fads for long-term good digestive health. These diets often classify foods as good or bad, and fruits are usually limited or eliminated on low-carbohydrate diet plans. Think of all of the fiber you're missing by foregoing an apple or a pear! The recipes here are rich in whole grains, and any diet with strict limits on the amount of carbohydrate you eat is not healthful for your digestive system.

If you're baffled by the words "seven-grain" or "multigrain" or even the notice "made with whole grain" on your product label, you're not alone. Here's how to find whole-grain, high-fiber foods.

- If the word "whole" is part of the first ingredient listed on the label, this is a whole-grain food. Other words you may see listed that are whole grains but won't use the word "whole" include barley, quinoa, buckwheat, oats, or brown rice.
- Next, you'll want to check the nutrition facts label for fiber. You'll find minimum guidelines for fiber for the foods used in these recipes on p 78, "Good Foods for Recipes."

Fiber in Prebiotic and Probiotic Foods

Most of us only get about half the fiber we need, and since this is one critical component of good digestive health, it's worth scouring the labels of your favorite foods for fiber. Our average daily intake is only about 15 grams per day, and we need a minimum of 25 grams per day. However, if you have a digestive disease and your physician has told you to limit your fiber intake, please follow the advice of your physician. In many cases, you will need to limit fiber for a short period of time, but always get permission from your physician to resume eating a fiber-rich diet.

There are two types of fiber: soluble and insoluble. The main difference is that soluble fiber dissolves in water and insoluble fiber doesn't. Foods rich in soluble fiber are also rich in prebiotic inulin and oligofructose, which feed the hungry probiotic bacteria in your colon. A University of California, Davis, study published in the *Journal of Nutrition* in 1999 noted that the chemical, biological, and physical properties of dietary fiber are linked with important activity in both the small and large intestine. The healthful properties of fiber include its ability to disperse in water, as well as adding bulk to your diet and contributing to fermentation in your colon. These actions help fiber perform an essential role in maintaining gastrointestinal health. Soluble fiber-rich carbohydrates, those that disperse in water, are more readily digested by the probiotic bacteria in your colon.

Soluble fiber also traps carbohydrates in your digestive system and slows absorption, causing a slower release of these sugars into the bloodstream. This is not only helpful to those with diabetes or pre-diabetes, but also it helps quell appetite and can assist with weight loss. Soluble fiber binds to cholesterol in your digestive tract, which helps to eliminate it before it can be absorbed and may lower your blood cholesterol level.

Insoluble fiber may help to excrete bile in the small intestine, making the way for probiotic bacteria to enter the colon alive, safe, and sound. Insoluble fiber is found in whole-wheat products and vegetables.

Desperately Seeking Soluble Fiber

Although both soluble and insoluble fiber are healthful for feeding your bacteria, soluble fiber is a little harder to get.

Some Foods High in Soluble Fiber

Food	Amount Soluble Fiber, grams
Prunes, 6 medium	3.0
Kidney beans, ½ cup (115 g)	2.0
Pinto beans, ½ cup (115 g)	2.0
Brussels sprouts, cooked, ½ cup (62 g)	2.0
Oat bran, dry, ⅓ cup (33 g)	2.0
Orange, 1 medium	1.8
Oatmeal, dry, ⅓ cup (27 g)	1.3
Apple, 1 medium	1.2
Broccoli, cooked, ½ cup (78 g)	1.1
Grapefruit, ½ medium	1.1
Spinach, cooked, ½ cup (90 g)	0.5
Brown rice, cooked, ½ cup (82 g)	0.4
Whole-wheat bread, 1 slice *	0.4
Grapes, 1 cup (150 g)	0.3
Zucchini, cooked, ½ cup (120 g)	0.2

*Check the label on your favorite whole-wheat bread. Some are higher in soluble fiber.

You can incorporate more soluble fiber-rich foods in your diet with a few substitutions:

* Have whole fruit instead of fruit juice.
* Toss ½ cup (115 g) of beans into your salad instead of ½ cup (15 g) of croutons.
* Instead of applesauce, eat apples with the peel.
* Instead of grits, have oatmeal for breakfast.

Gluten-Free…Yet Fiber-Full

Getting enough fiber can be a challenge if you're following a gluten-free diet. Gluten is a protein found in wheat, rye, barley, and some oats. Imagine having to consider every bite of food you put in your mouth. If you're avoiding gluten, every cookie, piece of bread, and dollop of salad dressing must be scrutinized. And by avoiding gluten, you may miss out on some fiber. The foods listed here will provide mostly insoluble fiber, but be sure to include soluble fiber from fruits and oats and oat fiber, if you can tolerate them, since this is the fiber that feeds your probiotic bacteria. Expand your choices and keep the fiber coming by checking out the latest healthful gluten-free choices, or try foods that are naturally gluten free.

Gluten-Free at the Grocery Store

The following products are listed with serving size and grams of fiber per serving in parentheses.

* Amy Lyn's Organic Flax Thins (Gluten-Free Crackers) (5 crackers, 7 g fiber)

- Bob's Red Mill Gluten-Free, Hearty, Whole-Grain Bread Mix (2 slices bread, 4 g fiber)
- Glutino Gluten-Free Flax Crackers, Tomato and Onion Flavor (8 crackers, 8 g fiber)
- Heartland's Finest Rotini (1 cup dry, 5 g fiber)
- Heartland's Finest Gluten-Free CerO's (1 cup, 3 g fiber)

Naturally Gluten-Free Foods
- Brown or wild rice
- Buckwheat pasta
- Corn
- Fresh fruit and vegetables
- Kasha
- Popcorn (air-popped or 94 percent reduced-fat microwave popcorn)
- Potatoes, sweet potatoes
- Quinoa

For the tastiest high-fiber baked goods, make your own cookies and muffins using flaxseed meal and buckwheat flour (Arrowhead Mills is one brand). These ingredients are available at some grocery stores, some health-food stores, and via mail order.

Too Much Sugar

The most preferred taste sensation is that for sweet foods. The word "sugar" conjures up an image of the sugar bowl sitting on your counter shelf, but that isn't the only type of sugar out there. The sugar that occurs naturally in milk is lactose, and the sugar in fruit is fructose. Many foods have some added sugar, sometimes when you least expect it. For example, soy milk has added sugar. And it's a good thing, since it would taste pretty bad and you wouldn't drink it otherwise! Sugar that is used to enhance nutrient-rich foods such as dried cranberries or soy milk is helping you pack more nutrition into your day in a very nice way. These recipes do have a little bit of added sugar, but not so much that it feeds your bad bacteria, allowing it to take over and kill off the probiotic bacteria.

According to the USDA, people who consume a diet high in sugar get less fiber. They also run short on calcium, folate, iron, magnesium, vitamin A, vitamin C, vitamin E, and zinc. And here's the icing on the cake, so to speak: These people also consume fewer fruits and vegetables. Sugar can also cause havoc during fermentation in your colon. It's speculated that bad bacteria prefer to feed on added sugars, causing overgrowth of bad versus good bacteria there.

Simple sugars, or monosaccharides, are made up of single-sugar molecules and have 4 calories per gram. Examples of simple sugars are glucose, fructose, and galactose. For some types of sweeteners, two of these simple sugars are joined together by a chemical bond and are called disaccharides. For example, table sugar is made from equal amounts of glucose and fructose. Starches and fiber are polysaccharides since they are made up of more than two simple sugars.

Fructose: a monosaccharide, or simple sugar found in agave nectar, fruits, honey, and root vegetables

Galactose: a monosaccharide found in milk products

Glucose: the sugar that is produced when you digest carbohydrates; your body's main source of energy

Lactose: the sugar found naturally in milk, it is a disaccharide composed of one galactose unit and one glucose unit. Many people cannot digest lactose, but probiotic bacteria can make the symptoms of lactose intolerance, including gas and bloating, more bearable.

Sucrose: commonly referred to as table sugar and composed of one glucose unit and one fructose unit

The Food and Drug Administration (FDA) has examined all sugars, including glucose, sucrose, high-fructose corn syrup, lactose, and many others. They've all been given the seal of approval. The FDA has determined that they are "generally recognized as safe" (GRAS). That means they have a proven track record of safety, based either on a history of use or on published scientific evidence, and can be freely used in food products.

High-Fructose Corn Syrup— Deadly or Not?

While you're eating for good digestive health, you can eat a little bit of added sugar. But many diet books and health advocacy groups warn against the health danger of consuming any foods with high-fructose corn syrup (HFCS). HFCS is the scapegoat for so many ills it wouldn't be prudent to list them all here. Is it possible that this sweetener is responsible for the obesity epidemic and a variety of diseases? After years of study, scientists say no.

HFCS has gotten kicked around recently, and because of all the media attention, it's become one of the most recognized ingredients on a food label. It shows up in such foods as yogurt and salad dressing. Here's the skinny from the scientific studies to date: The bashing of HFCS is primarily around the fact that there are more obese people now than ever before. The debate started with regards to soda drinking. People drink a lot of soda, and sodas are high in HFCS. Soda is considered a major factor contributing to the obesity crisis. But HFCS in soda can't take the brunt of the blame. If soft-drink manufacturers made soda from white cane sugar, and people drank just as much as they did before, *they'd gain the same amount of weight.* Both HFCS and sugar contribute the same number of calories. And that's not all they have in common. Both white cane sugar and HFCS are disaccharides made from molecules of fructose and glucose. Most scientists believe the body doesn't differentiate between HFCS and white cane sugar.

There is some research that indicates that fructose alone (used as a sweetener in this manner) may have more obesity-inducing qualities than HFCS, white cane sugar, or corn syrup. But pure fructose is not a common additive to sweeten our foods. Corn syrup, for example, is all glucose with no fructose at all. There are two different versions of HFCS commonly used right now: one that is 42 percent fructose and 53 percent glucose, and one that is 55 percent fructose and 42 percent glucose (both versions contain a small fraction of other sugars). Both versions act similarly to white cane sugar in your body, not inciting disease or causing obesity all by itself.

The health professionals at the Center for Science in the Public Interest (CSPI)—also known as the "food police" and the home of the *Nutrition Action Healthletter*, one of the most well-respected health education magazines around—agree that HFCS is a safe sweetener. Of course, it's not recommended to seek out HFCS or foods with lots of added sugar, but if they're added in small quantities to foods that are otherwise healthful, go ahead and enjoy them. But let's take HFCS out of the spotlight. For your very best digestive health, limit your intake of sugary foods to between 100 and 300 calories per day. Here's

how to figure out your discretionary calories, according to the USDA's Center for Nutrition Policy and Promotion. (See right.)

What Are Discretionary Calories?

You need a certain number of calories to keep your body functioning and provide energy

---

HOW TO DETERMINE YOUR DISCRETIONARY CALORIES

For example, assume your calorie budget is 2,000 calories per day. Of these calories, you need to spend at least 1,735 calories for essential nutrients, if you choose foods without added fat and sugar. That leaves you with 265 discretionary calories. You may use these on "luxury" versions of the foods in each group, such as higher-fat meat or sweetened cereal. Or, you can spend them on sweets, sauces, or beverages. Many people overspend their discretionary calorie allowance, choosing more added fats, sugars, and alcohol than their budget allows.

You can use your discretionary calorie allowance to:

- eat more foods from any food group than the food guide recommends
- eat higher calorie forms of foods—those that contain solid fats or added sugars—such as biscuits, cheese, sausage, sweetened cereal, sweetened yogurt, and whole milk
- add fats or sweeteners to foods, such as butter, salad dressings, sauces, sugar, and syrup
- eat or drink items that are mostly fats, caloric sweeteners, and/or alcohol, such as candy, soda, wine, and beer

Reprinted with permission from the USDA Center for Nutrition Policy and Promotion, 2007

for physical activities. Think of calories like money you have to spend. Each person has a total calorie "budget." This budget can be divided into "essentials" and "extras."

With a financial budget, the essentials are items like rent and food. The extras are things like movies and vacations. In a calorie budget, the essentials are the minimum calories required to meet your nutrient needs. By selecting the lowest fat and no-sugar-added forms of foods in each food group, you would make the best nutrient "buys." Depending on the foods you choose, you may be able to spend more calories than the amount required to meet your nutrient needs. These calories are the "extras" that can be used on luxuries like solid fats, added sugars, and alcohol, or on more food from any food group. They are your "discretionary calories."

Each person has an allowance for some discretionary calories. But many people use up the allowance before lunch! Most discretionary calorie allowances are very small, between 100 and 300 calories, especially for those who are not physically active. For many people, the discretionary calorie allowance is totally used up by the foods they choose in each food group, such as higher-fat meats, cheeses, whole milk, or sweetened bakery products.

Put the Brakes on Dietary Fat

Some of the fats you eat may fit into this discretionary category, but for the very best digestive health and the safest environment for your probiotic bacteria, choose a low-fat diet and make sure that most of the fats you choose are healthful omega-3s and unsaturated fats including nuts, avocado, tahini (sesame seed paste), hummus, olives, and seeds.

USDA LIMITS FOR DIETARY FAT CONTENT

What constitutes a high-fat diet? According to the USDA, any diet containing 30 percent or more of daily calories from fat is considered a "high-fat" diet. To maintain the best possible intestinal health, try to put a cap on your daily fat intake at 30 percent of calories.

Calorie Intake	Maximum Daily Fat
1,600	53 grams
1,700	57 grams
1,800	60 grams
1,900	63 grams
2,000	67 grams
2,100	70 grams
2,200	73 grams
2,300	77 grams
2,400	80 grams
2,500	83 grams
2,600	87 grams
2,700	90 grams
2,800	93 grams

A diet high in fat can exclude fiber, which is critical for feeding your probiotic bacteria. Unhealthy fats, including saturated and trans fats, are particularly harmful for your digestive function and the viability of your good bacteria. The bacteria in your colon help produce secondary bile acids there, and they break down the bile salts necessary to digest fat. When the bacteria are overwhelmed with too much fat, this is not a smooth process, and if the bacteria don't get fed enough fiber, they won't survive. So keep your bacteria alive by following these upper limits for fat grams per day.

Control Intake of Saturated and Trans Fats

Experts say your saturated fat intake should be limited to less than 10 percent of total calories. The American Heart Association has recently set the bar even lower at 7 percent of total calories, which means if you consume 2,000 daily calories, you should limit saturated fat to 16 grams per day. Saturated fats are found in the following foods: the skin of poultry, whole dairy products (butter, regular cheese, whole milk, regular ice cream, sour cream, and cream cheese), low-fat versions of dairy (1 or 2 percent milk and low-fat cheese, sour cream, and ice cream), and fatty cuts of meat like ground beef. Those 16 grams can quickly add up: a slice of cheese may have up to 6 grams, and only a half-cup of ice cream can pack 10 grams. Small amounts of saturated fat are found in all oils as well, so you'll have

to account for some of this fat in even your healthiest food choices. The foods included in these recipes may include some saturated fat; it's not possible to avoid it altogether!

With the appearance of trans fats on nutrition facts labels in January 2006, manufacturers started reducing their use of trans fats. The recommendation is to limit trans fats to 1 percent of total calories. That's 1.5 g on a 1,500-calorie diet. Trans fats are mainly found in foods containing partially hydrogenated vegetable oil, such as cookies, pie crusts, chips, and other snack foods, so try to limit your intake of these or choose trans fat-free versions.

Even though food labels are now required to list trans fats, they may not accurately reflect the food's true amount. There are plenty of foods on the shelves packing a lot more trans fat than meets the eye. Some labels may report "0 grams trans fat," but the FDA allows manufacturers to claim 0 grams trans fat if the product has up to 0.49 grams. A few servings of foods with 0.49 grams of trans fats adds up very quickly. Even if you don't think trans fats are in a food, always check the ingredients list for the words "partially hydrogenated" associated with any type of oil. If this type of fat is listed, see where it falls in the lineup of ingredients. The sooner it shows up in the list, the more likely it is that your food has enough trans fat that you will want to swap it for another food that doesn't list any partially hydrogenated oils.

Omega-6 Fatty Acids

These essential fatty acids are important to get in your diet, but Americans get about ten times the amount they need in any given day. The composition of these fats is not as health-promoting as that of omega-3 fats. Omega-6 fats are made from arachidonic acid (AA) and linoleic acid (LA). These fats promote inflammation and disease, so watch your intake of corn, cottonseed, safflower, soybean, sunflower, and vegetable oils (and foods made with these oils); meats, including organ meats; and other animal-based foods. The recipes in this book will guide the way to good digestive health with meatless choices as well as ample healthful fats.

Omega-3 Fatty Acids

Since you're controlling your fat intake to help better manage your intestinal flora, you might as well eat the best possible fats. The health benefits of omega-3 fats are verified by many clinical trials and population studies. The anti-inflammatory properties of these fats protect against heart disease, inhibit cholesterol buildup in your arteries, lower blood pressure, and lower blood triglyceride levels. These super fats are shown to help prevent and improve the symptoms of diabetes, arthritis, and cancer. People who consume a diet rich in omega-3 fats also have a lower risk of suffering from major depression. Omega-3 fats don't disrupt the bacterial balance in your digestive tract like saturated, trans, or omega-6 fats do.

Omega-3 fatty acids are available in three forms: alpha-linolenic acid (ALA), technically a pre-form for omega-3 fats; eicosapentaenoic acid (EPA); and docosahexaenoic acid (DHA). Dietary sources of ALA include beans, canola oil, eggs, flaxseed oil and seeds, pumpkin seeds, soybeans, tofu, and walnuts. There are even eggs available that are rich in ALA (these are from chickens fed a diet high in ALA). EPA and DHA are available in seafood such as albacore tuna, herring, lake trout, mackerel, salmon, sardines, and many other fish.

Most health experts recommend about 1 gram daily of EPA and DHA (or eating the recommended fish three times per week) and 1.6 grams ALA for women and 1.1 grams for men daily (2 tablespoons of walnuts has about 1.1 grams ALA, and 1 tablespoon of canola oil has 1.3 grams, so this is pretty easy to get).

Vitamin B12—A Special Vitamin

Vitamin B12 is naturally found in foods that come from animals, including dairy products, eggs, fish, meat, and poultry. These foods are a source of vitamin B12 because the animals they come from consume foods that are contaminated with bacteria that produce vitamin B12. We need vitamin B12 to maintain a healthy nervous system, to produce red blood cells, and to synthesize DNA, our genetic material. Since vitamin B12 comes from animal foods, it becomes harder to get with these recipes.

How Vitamin B12 Is Absorbed

We absorb vitamin B12 by a complex process. Vitamin B12 is bound to the protein in animal foods. When these foods are eaten and reach the stomach, stomach acid and enzymes separate vitamin B12 from food proteins, and vitamin B12 attaches to other proteins called R proteins. In the small intestine, vitamin B12 is freed from the R proteins and binds to intrinsic factor, a protein produced by stomach cells. Binding to intrinsic factor allows vitamin B12 to be absorbed by the body through receptors on the surface of the small intestine. Vitamin B12 can also be absorbed by passive diffusion, but only a very small percentage of vitamin B12 is absorbed passively.

For us to absorb vitamin B12 from food, the digestive system—including the stomach, pancreas, and small intestine—needs to be functioning properly. Problems with any of these organs could lead to a vitamin B12 deficiency. The bacteria that reside in our digestive tract can also affect our absorption of vitamin B12.

How Much Vitamin B12 Do We Need?

The current Recommended Dietary Allowance (RDA) of vitamin B12 for adults is 2.4 micrograms per day. Women who are pregnant or lactating have a slightly higher RDA. In the United States, the average intake of vitamin B12 is about 1.5 to 2 times the RDA, and most people who eat foods from animals do not have trouble meeting the RDA. No known problems are associated with consuming high amounts of vitamin B12.

Vegans and adults over age 50 are advised to consume fortified foods or supplements containing vitamin B12 to meet their needs. Foods fortified with vitamin B12 include some fortified cereals, soy milks, and meat substitutes.

Up to 30 percent of adults over age 50 don't absorb food-bound vitamin B12 well due to an insufficient amount of stomach acid, digestive enzymes, or intrinsic factor. In the case of fortified food and supplements, stomach acid and digestive enzymes are not needed to detach vitamin B12 from protein because vitamin B12 in supplemental form is not bound to protein. If supplemental vitamin B12 is taken in a large enough dose, a significant amount can also be absorbed through passive diffusion, thus bypassing the usual method of vitamin B12 absorption.

Deficiency of vitamin B12 leads to pernicious anemia, gastrointestinal disorders, and neurological abnormalities. Because vitamin B12 is stored in the body, mainly in the liver, a person who is consuming an insufficient amount of vitamin B12 may not show deficiency symptoms for several years.

Vegan Sources of Vitamin B12

Because natural food sources of vitamin B12 are from animals, vegans risk developing a vitamin B12 deficiency. The current consensus is that any vitamin B12 present in plant foods is likely to be unavailable to humans, and plant foods should therefore not be relied upon as source of vitamin B12. To avoid a vitamin B12 deficiency, it is recommended that vegans eat foods that are fortified with vitamin B12 or take a supplement containing vitamin B12.

While nutritional yeasts (Red Star is a reliable brand) are often considered a source of vitamin B12 for vegans, not all nutritional yeasts contain vitamin B12. It is important for vegans to read product labels of fortified foods carefully, and ideally, they should not rely solely on one type of fortified food to meet their vitamin B12 needs. Vegans might be able to enhance their vitamin B12 status by influencing their intestinal flora with probiotics.

Probiotics and Vitamin B12

Bacteria in the human intestinal tract have been found to produce vitamin B12. However, most studies have concluded that the vast majority, if not all, of these vitamin B12-producing bacteria reside in the large intestine. Because we can only absorb vitamin B12 through our small intestine, vitamin B12 produced in the large intestine is too far along our digestive tract for us to absorb, and it is therefore excreted.

There is an ongoing controversy about whether intestinal bacteria could provide enough vitamin B12 to meet the nutritional requirements of a person who does not consume any vitamin B12 from foods or supplements. Several researchers have suggested that if a small amount of the right strains of bacteria is introduced into the small intestine, this could significantly improve a person's vitamin B12 status.

On the other hand, overgrowth of bacteria in the small intestine has been found in some cases to contribute to a vitamin B12 deficiency. Certain bacteria take up vitamin B12 for their own use and therefore do not allow the body to absorb it. Vegans should be sure to obtain an adequate amount of vitamin B12 from fortified foods and supplements. As the field continues to expand, probiotics may be developed to provide significant amounts of vitamin B12 to vegans and others who need to optimize their vitamin B12 status.

Choose the Right Multi

It's important to consider taking a multivitamin/mineral supplement (multi) to get adequate vitamin B12 while following your prebiotic- and probiotic-rich meatless diet. Many health experts recommend taking a multi; even with a healthful diet day in and day out, it's hard to get every last milligram of every vitamin and mineral to meet your minimum daily needs. Your age, sex, and environment also set your personal bar higher or lower for some vitamins and minerals.

Several studies show that multis are helpful for improving micronutrient status and reducing the risk for several chronic diseases in the elderly. One long-term study showed less progression of age-related macular degeneration in people taking beta-carotene, vitamins C and E, and zinc.

When choosing the right multi for you, look for more of these vitamins that you may run short on, even with the most healthful diet:

Vitamin D Men and women age 50 and older may benefit from vitamin D supplementation. People with dark skin are also at risk for vitamin D deficiency since they need to spend more time in the sun to synthesize it. Our need for vitamin D increases as we get older, and since the skin is less able to synthesize vitamin D from sunlight as we age, it may be wise to take a multi with vitamin D. For adults age 51 to 70, the requirement is 400 IU (international units) per day, and at age 71 and older, the need increases to 600 IU per day.

Vitamin K The daily value for vitamin K is 120 mcg (micrograms), but research suggests that people need more to reduce the risk of hip fracture and improve bone density. A multi can help make up the difference.

If you take an anti-coagulant, ask your doctor if you can take supplemental vitamin K. Your doctor can monitor you with International Normalized Ratio (INR). If you want to take a multi with vitamin K, INR management is essential. If your doctor isn't using INR, don't take any supplemental vitamin K.

Pay close attention to the following vitamins and minerals since too much can be a problem for some people:

Iron Look for a maximum of 10 mg (milligrams) of iron in your multi. Too much iron can put those of us with a tendency toward iron overload (a condition called hemochromatosis) at risk. Pre-menopausal women may need a bit more; about 18 mg is adequate.

Vitamin A Your maximum intake from a supplement should be 4,000 IU of vitamin A. A diet rich in vegetables, which you'll find in these recipes, can provide all you need, so don't use this as a minimum amount. Too much supplemental vitamin A can increase your risk of hip fracture, liver abnormalities, and birth defects.

Vitamin E Look for around 100 IU of vitamin E. Too much supplemental vitamin E is not necessary and doesn't decrease your risk for cancer or sudden cardiac events, as previously believed.

You may need to take a separate supplement to get enough of these minerals:

Calcium and Magnesium These minerals have a little more mass, so you won't be able to pack much calcium and magnesium into a multi. Try to get what you need from your diet or take a separate mineral supplement if advised by your doctor or licensed nutritionist to do so.

Multi Savvy

Select the best multi using the following guidelines. For each of the vitamins and minerals listed below, look for 100 percent of the daily value. Always store your bottle in a cool, dry place and honor the expiration date.

Vitamin B1 (thiamin)
Vitamin B2 (riboflavin)
Vitamin B3 (niacin)
Vitamin B12
Vitamin C
Vitamin D
Folic acid

For the following vitamins and minerals, here's how to choose:

Vitamin or Mineral	Amount (Look for at Least)
Chromium	35 mcg
Copper	0.9 mg
Magnesium	100 mg, and no more than 350 mg
Selenium	50 mcg
Zinc	11 mg, and no more than 23 mg

Vitamin or Mineral	Amount (Look for No More Than)
Vitamin A	4,000 IU
Vitamin E	100 IU
Iron	18 mg
Phosphorus	350 mg
Vitamin B6	100 mg
Beta-carotene	15,000 IU

Choose Based on Your Age and Sex			
Vitamin or Mineral	Premeno-pausal Women	Men Under 50	Age 50+ (Men and Women)
Iron	18 mg	10 mg	10 mg
Vitamin K	25 mcg	25 mcg	10 mcg
Vitamin B12	6 mcg	6 mcg	12 mcg

The nutrient-rich foods in your prebiotic and probiotic recipes make it easy to manage good digestive health. The resulting bacterial balance from this healthful diet will help reduce your risk for disease and improve your overall immunity. Your lifestyle also has a big impact on your digestive health, including gastric bypass surgery to manage obesity, smoking, alcohol, and physical activity. Clean living does have advantages for the best digestive health!

CHAPTER FIVE

Living Well for Digestive Health

Think of someone you know with an unhealthy lifestyle. Maybe they smoke, drink too much alcohol, eat a terrible diet, or don't exercise. You can see it in their waistline, or they constantly complain that they're tired. Perhaps they struggle with simple things like walking up a short flight of stairs. Overall, they seem to be trudging through life rather than living it. If you can spot someone this unhealthy at a glance from the outside, can you imagine what's happening on the *inside*?

Unhealthy habits can take their toll on your digestive system. Factors such as alcohol, lack of exercise, bariatric surgery for obesity, and smoking all have a profound impact on the bacterial balance in your digestive tract. When your bacteria are out of balance, it can cause improper absorption of nutrients, constipation, diarrhea, poor immunity, and disease. Here is the impact that these vices can have on your well being.

Last Call for Alcohol

One serving of alcohol is 1½ ounces of hard liquor, 4 ounces of wine, 12 ounces of beer, or a 10-ounce wine cooler. Chronic abuse of alcohol is a big problem for your digestive bacterial health. A 2003 study published in *Best Practice and Research, Clinical Gastroenterology* found that consumption of large quantities of alcoholic beverages leads to disturbances in the intestinal absorption of nutrients, including several vitamins. Alcohol abuse inhibits the absorption of sodium and water in the colon and can cause chronic diarrhea. If you drink too much alcohol, this can cause duodenal erosions, bleeding, and mucosal injury. As a result, many alcoholics have bad bacterial overgrowth in the small intestine, which may contribute to functional abnormalities of this part of the gut. The mucosal damage caused by alcohol increases the permeability of the gut to larger molecules, and this facilitates the transfer of endotoxin (the potentially toxic cell membrane of a bacterial cell) and other bacterial toxins from the gut lumen to the portal blood (through your liver), risking overexposure of the liver to toxins and increasing the risk of liver injury. Ultimately, this can impair immunity.

Most people make the connection between too much alcohol and poor liver function. In fact, the most common cause of liver problems is malnutrition related to alcohol abuse. All the functions of your liver can be adversely affected by alcohol and bacterial invasion.

Functions of the Liver

- Filters the blood
- Makes bile, which is transported to the intestines to help digest fat
- Processes and hooks or attaches fats (such as cholesterol) to carriers
- Stores sugars, transports them, and saves energy
- Makes protein for clotting blood
- Metabolizes medications (for example, barbiturates, sedatives, and amphetamines)
- Stores vitamins and minerals including iron, copper, vitamins A and D, and some B vitamins
- Makes albumin, which is critical for regulating fluid transport in the blood and kidneys
- Helps break down and recycle red blood cells

It's plain to see why you'd want to keep your liver healthy! Just one serving of the wrong type of alcoholic beverage can cause a problem with bacterial balance. Beer; champagne; cocktails made with gin, vermouth or vodka; red or white wine; and sherry are classified as fermented alcoholic beverages, which can stimulate a potent release of gastrin. This can cause a problem if you are infected with *Heliobacter pylori* (*H. pylori*), a bad bacterium; when gastrin is released in the stomach, it can break through the mucous lining of the stomach or duodenum, causing an ulcer.

Even a small amount of any type of alcohol can accelerate gastric motility, and this can decrease the exposure of your good bacteria to the prebiotics that feed your probiotic bacteria and help them flourish. Over time, this can cause an imbalance of bad over good bacteria in your colon. Endotoxemia and liver injury as a result of alcohol abuse can be helped with probiotic bacteria *Lactobacillus* species GG.

Obesity and Gastric Bypass Surgery

More and more people are turning to bariatric surgery such gastric banding, Roux-en-Y gastric bypass, and other types of banding and gastric bypass procedures that promote weight loss. There are many theories about the obesity crisis. Maybe we're heavier than ever before due to inactivity or huge portions of food, and it's probably a little bit of both, but one method to facilitate weight loss for people with a Body Mass Index (BMI) of 40 or greater is gastric bypass surgery. Since these procedures involve manipulation of the digestive tract, there is an impact on intestinal bacteria. In fact, it's speculated that one of the mechanisms by which people lose weight via gastric bypass surgery is through gastric inflammation and *H. pylori* infection following the surgery. A 2006 study published in *Obesity Surgery: The Official Journal of the American Society for Bariatric Surgery and of the Obesity Surgery Society of Australia and New Zealand* confirmed that this infection and inflammation play a significant role in the amount of weight lost through laparoscopic vertical banded gastroplasty. But upsetting your gastrointestinal system may not be the safest way to lose weight.

According to a 2007 study published in the *Journal of Clinical Pathology*, following Roux-en-Y gastric bypass surgery there is a loss of gastric-acid-mediated protection against bad bacteria entering the digestive system through the mouth. Probiotic bacteria need to survive the harsh environment of digestion, including exposure to gastric acid in the stomach, but gastric acid serves another purpose as well: to kill bad bacteria there. After gastric bypass surgery, researchers found an increased secretion of human defensin 5 (HD-5) and an increase in HD-5 expression in the jejunal mucosa (this is an inflammatory reaction to the bad bacteria), which is likely due to the bad microbes introduced through the mouth that aren't being killed by gastric acid. These bad bacteria have potential to flourish in the colon, overtaking the good bacteria and upsetting the balance.

According to a study published in *Kidney International*, Roux-en-Y gastric bypass surgery can have an impact on oxalate formation in the urine, a potentially serious complication increasing the incidence of kidney stone formation. The study found that probiotic use can positively manipulate the gastrointestinal flora and reduce urinary oxalate kidney stone formation in post–gastric bypass patients.

Gastric bypass surgery patients can have disturbing side effects including diarrhea, foul flatulence, and abdominal cramping. The American Society for Bariatric Surgery recommends a course of probiotics (a course usually means two to three weeks of daily use), specifically *L. acidophilus*, to help alleviate these symptoms. Gastric bypass hardly seems like the best answer for every morbidly obese person; eating a diet rich in these probiotic and prebiotic foods can help control calorie intake since they're high in fiber, low in fat, and very satisfying. During weight loss, studies also show that both prebiotic and probiotic foods are instrumental in alleviating the constipation that can result from a low-calorie diet.

Smoking and Your Digestive Health

According to the American Heart Association (AHA), smoking is the most preventable cause of death in the United States. Smokers are two to three times more likely to die from heart disease than nonsmokers, and smoking is linked to a poor outcome from nearly every health angle, including digestive health.

Smoking is a causative factor for bladder cancer. Probiotic yogurt containing *L. casei* is beneficial for prevention of bladder cancer in smokers, according to a review published in *Der Urologe*, a German medical journal, in 2007. Milk containing *L. casei* was given to smokers in a study published in *Preventive Medicine* in 2005, and the results showed this was effective at restoring natural killer (NK) cell activity. NK cells are a type of white blood cell that contains granules with enzymes that can kill tumor cells or microbial cells.

Smoking has been identified as a risk factor for Crohn's disease. Yet strangely enough, for those suffering from ulcerative colitis, those who have never smoked or formerly smoked show an *increased* risk of ulcers. It's not recommended that people who suffer from chronic ulcerative colitis *start* smoking, but the experimental use of nicotine patches does seem to offer some relief of intestinal symptoms. Further studies with larger patient populations are needed to clarify this treatment.

H. pylori is a bacterium that can cause bloating, gastritis, heartburn, nausea, and ulcers in the stomach or intestine. Smoking can be irritating to the stomach and is known to aggravate *H. pylori* infection. *H. pylori* can be treated with antibiotics, and probiotic bacteria are helpful to alleviate symptoms. The probiotic bacteria can survive combination therapy with antibiotics. The types of probiotic bacteria that are helpful include *Lactobacillus rhamnosus* GG, *L. rhamnosus* LC705, *Bifidobacterium breve* Bb99, and *Propionibacterium freudenreichii*ssp. shermanii JS.

How to Stop Smoking

There are some great resources to help you quit smoking for good. Choose your method for quitting carefully so you can make smoking a thing of the past. In 2002, a *New England Journal of Medicine* study tracked over 3,000 smokers who were poised to quit smoking. According to researchers at the University of California at San Diego, a full 21 percent of smokers who took advantage of counseling via a "quitline" (a toll-free phone number with trained counselors to help) kicked the habit, versus only 10 percent of those who didn't get the counseling. One of the reasons that quitlines work is that the counselors can, in some cases, offer optimal support because they're objective, they don't have high expectations, and they are not emotionally involved with the person trying to quit smoking.

Another option is to visit the AHA website (www.americanheart.org) and click on "Healthy Lifestyle," then "Smoking and Cardiovascular Disease," and finally "Stop Smoking: Resources and Tools for Quitting."

Exercise for Digestive Health

Keep moving and you'll keep your digestive balance on track. Exercise can stimulate peristalsis, which helps maintain bowel regularity. Constipation is a risk factor for overgrowth of bad bacteria in the colon. In disabled and elderly adults, small-bowel bacterial overgrowth is more prevalent than in active, healthy adults. In other studies, physical inactivity (measured as the number of steps taken daily) in elderly individuals is associated with decreased intestinal transit time, constipation, and small-bowel bacterial overgrowth. This overgrowth is sometimes associated with either constipation or diarrhea. When the overgrowth is severe and goes on for months or years, the bacteria may interfere with the digestion and/or absorption of food, and deficiencies of vitamins and minerals may develop (see p 14, "The Vitamin Connection"). This overgrowth can also cause weight loss, body aches, or fatigue.

Your Diamond Exercise Plan

When you structure your exercise plan, think of the four sides of a diamond to include everything you need. These four components work together to give you a balanced, comprehensive program.

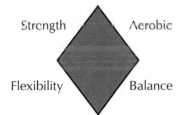

Strength   Aerobic

Flexibility   Balance

Balance problems plague many of us as we get older. Falling and breaking a bone or causing an injury is one of the biggest fears that older adults have. This makes people a little more timid about moving for exercise. According

to the American College of Sports Medicine (ACSM) guidelines, your well-rounded exercise plan should include strength, flexibility, aerobic, and balance components.

Strength These exercises build muscle mass and strength to help prevent the effects of arthritis and to prevent injuries due to lifting and carrying heavy objects in daily life. Weight-bearing exercises can help combat the effects of osteoporosis.

Sample exercises include:

1. Biceps curl with a hand weight (for animated directions on this and other strength exercises please visit the National Institute on Aging website at www.niapublications.org/exercisebook/chapter4_strength.htm)
2. Chair stand (stand up out of a chair with arms crossed over the chest)

Perform one set of 8 to 15 repetitions of each exercise. Choose 8 to 10 exercises minimum per workout covering all major muscle groups and do the routine 2 to 3 times per week. Wait at least 48 hours in between strength workouts to allow your muscles to repair tiny tears that occur during muscle-building exercise.

Flexibility These exercises help keep muscles loose so they are not easily strained during daily activities and workouts. They can also reduce muscle tension due to prolonged sitting and other periods of inactivity.

Sample exercises include:

1. Seated hamstring stretch (for directions on this and other flexibility exercises please visit www.niapublications.org/exercisebook/chapter4_stretching.htm)
2. Standing calf stretch for keeping the ankles flexible, which can allow you to walk more freely and move more easily

For each stretching exercise, perform 2 to 4 repetitions and hold each stretch 15 to 30 seconds to a point of tightness, without discomfort. Do stretching exercises a minimum of 2 times per week, but ideally 5 times per week.

Aerobic These exercises increase the HDL-cholesterol level (good cholesterol), lower blood pressure, reduce risk of obesity (which, in turn, prevents strain on the joints), and can give you the endurance to accomplish daily tasks with greater ease.

Sample exercises include:

1. Outdoor activity, such as walking, hiking, tennis, volleyball
2. Indoor activity, such as using a treadmill, dancing

Perform aerobic exercises 3 to 5 times per week for 20 to 60 minutes of continuous or intermittent activity (such as 10-minute bouts that accumulate throughout the day).

Balance These exercises help reduce falls, which is important for lowering risk for fractures associated with osteoporosis, and may help you prevent falls and accidents from recreational activities such as skiing or tennis.

Sample exercises include:

1. Any type of dance class (tango, ballroom, salsa)
2. Standing on a balance board (also called a wobble board)

Physical therapist Z. Altug, M.S., C.S.C.S., recommends "doing simple balance exercises (such as single leg toe raises without holding on to anything) at least 2 to 3 times per week, but for optimal balance, do these 5 to 7 times per week."

It's tempting to try to bypass doing the right things for good health. So many of us sit too much, can't get into the swing of a regular exercise routine, or don't know how to start exercising safely. Too much fat, lots of sugary foods, and too much alcohol are a big part of our celebrations. Eating the right foods and living a healthy lifestyle sometimes seem so far out of reach. But when you see how your body works in concert with healthful foods for improving digestive bacterial balance, and how exercise helps to regulate transit time of food and waste through your digestive tract, it can help you embrace these habits to improve immunity and reduce your risk for disease.

CHAPTER SIX

Cooking with Probiotic and Prebiotic Recipes for Digestive Health

The key to eating healthfully is to find foods that you like and that are easy to prepare. The dishes here include probiotic and prebiotic foods that you can whip up quickly and easily. The list of ingredients for each dish is minimal, and the flavors combine to make a satisfying, tasty main course or side dish, with suggestions to round out your meal and make it complete.

Choosing ingredients that meet the prebiotic and probiotic nutrient guidelines can be a challenge, so we've included a chart for commercially available foods you'll want to have on hand. Kefir is one such food, but many people prefer to make their own, so this begins our recipe section.

Feel-Good Kefir

Kefir is the flagship probiotic product, one of the first foods eaten with live bacteria cultures for health benefits. The name kefir loosely translates to "good feeling." It's a fermented milk drink that has recently gained popularity with media attention on the health benefits of probiotics. If you want to try kefir, and you're not comfortable relying on a ready-made version of kefir for your recipes, you may want to make your own. This may also be your best option if you can't find kefir on your grocery shelf. Making kefir at home is fairly straightforward, but the process involves some waiting time.

Time for an Oil Change

You can add flavor to foods by experimenting with the many gourmet oils now available. The oils listed here have the right kind of fat and will give you big flavor for just a few calories. You can also try oil sprays. They're a great way to control the fat content of your favorite dishes and help you maintain a lower-fat diet for the best digestive health. Use the spray to lightly coat your food without adding many extra calories or a heavy taste. Some of the flavored sprays now available include olive oil, grapeseed oil, and canola oil.

Oils add unique flavor to your dishes. Just like fresh herbs, some enhance the flavor of your salad or cold dish and some are great for cooking. Look for the words "expeller-pressed" on the label, which means the oil has been extracted in the healthiest way possible to preserve nutrients and taste. All oils should be stored in a cool, dark place, but not in the refrigerator, please! This will cause a cloudy, unpleasant-looking product. (See page 81.)

Good Foods for Recipes

These foods have been selected because they contain the right amounts of fat and fiber, resulting in the best nutritional benefit. If you can't find the brand mentioned, substitute another food with similar nutritional value. The chart lists soluble fiber where appropriate and notes the percentages of calcium and vitamin D in the milks, since these are important nutrients for good health.

Commercial Foods	Nutrition Facts
High-fiber snack bar, such as Kashi TLC Granola Bar	One bar: 140–180 calories, 5 g fat, 0.5 g saturated fat, 0 g trans fat, 0 mg cholesterol, 21 g carbohydrate, 5 g protein, 100 mg sodium, 4 g fiber (1 g soluble fiber)
Frozen whole-grain, high-fiber waffles	Two waffles: 170 calories, 3 g fat, 0 g saturated fat, 0 g trans fat, 0 mg cholesterol, 33 g carbohydrate, 8 g protein, 330 mg sodium, 6 g fiber
High-fiber, whole-grain cereal	One serving: 170 calories, 2 g fat, 0 g saturated fat, 0 g trans fat, 0 mg cholesterol, 43 g carbohydrate, 5 g protein, 130 mg sodium, 12 g fiber (1 g soluble fiber)
Nonfat plain soy milk	One cup (235 ml): 70 calories, 0 g fat, 0 g saturated fat, 0 g trans fat, 0 mg cholesterol, 10 g carbohydrate, 6 g protein, 105 mg sodium, 0.5 g fiber, 250 mg calcium, 200 IU vitamin D
Nonfat (skim) cow's milk	One cup (235 ml): 83 calories, 0 g fat, 0 g saturated fat, 0 g trans fat, 4.9 mg cholesterol, 12 g carbohydrate, 8.3 g protein, 103 mg sodium, 0 g fiber, 306 mg calcium, 100 IU vitamin D
Low-fat goat's milk	One cup (235 ml): 89 calories, 2.4 g fat, 1.5 g saturated fat, 0 g trans fat, 8.4 mg cholesterol, 9.4 g carbohydrate, 7.4 g protein, 100 mg sodium, 0 g fiber, 268 mg calcium, 100 IU vitamin D
Whole-wheat crackers, such as Wasa Multigrain Crispbread	One serving: 90 calories, 0 g fat, 0 g saturated fat, 0 g trans fat, 0 mg cholesterol, 20 g carbohydrate, 4 g protein, 100 mg sodium, 4 g fiber
Pasta sauce	One half cup (125 g): 60 calories, 1 g fat, 0 g saturated fat, 0 g trans fat, 0 mg cholesterol, 10 g carbohydrate, 2 g protein, 390 mg sodium, 2 g fiber
Whole-grain wrap, such as Flatout Soft Wrap Multi-Grain	One wrap: 100 calories, 2.5 g fat, 0 g saturated fat, 0 g trans fat, 0 mg cholesterol, 17 g carbohydrate, 9 g protein, 380 mg sodium, 8 g fiber
Margarine, light, trans-fatfree	One tablespoon (14 g): 37 calories, 5 g fat, 1 g saturated fat, 0 g trans fat, 0 mg cholesterol, 0 g carbohydrate, 0 g protein, 85 mg sodium, 0 g fiber
Whole-wheat bread	One slice: 80 calories, 1 g fat, 0 g saturated fat, 0 g trans fat, 0 mg cholesterol, 18 g carbohydrate, 0 g protein, 170 mg sodium, 3 g fiber

MAKE YOUR OWN KEFIR

The easiest way to make kefir is to regularly replenish your ongoing supply of kefir milk, so follow these instructions if you find that making kefir at home agrees with you. If you're just starting out, you'll need to order kefir cultures. Pay special attention to how they are shipped, requesting the most prompt delivery you can afford. Don't hesitate to ask questions about the product (see p 26, "Four Questions").

To create a new batch of kefir, follow steps 2 through 10. If you are replenishing your supply, begin with a two- to three-day-old quart of kefir standing on the kitchen counter, and start with step 1.

1. First, make sure it tastes like you expect it to taste! The taste of your kefir will determine whether or not you'll use it, so don't discount this important first step.

2. Choose your milk carefully. Goat's milk is commonly chosen to make kefir. Full-fat goat's milk has too much saturated fat, so choose low-fat or nonfat milk. Set out your one-quart milk jar.

3. The kefir cultures you use will be a grain-like product. Strain your kefir grains by pouring them through a strainer into a bowl.

4. Squeeze some of the remaining liquid from the kefir grains by pressing against them with a small spoon.

5. Clean off the kefir grains by rinsing them with distilled water, purchased in bottles at the grocery store. Shift the grains around in the strainer to be sure that every last kefir grain gets a shower. Rinse for no less than two minutes and don't be tempted to use tap water—the chlorine can be harmful to kefir grains. Set the timer if necessary.

6. Leave a bit of room at the top of the milk jar to allow space for adding the kefir grains. Add about ³/₄ cup of kefir grains to a quart of fresh low-fat or nonfat goat's milk. Your kefir grains may multiply, so if you have more than ³/₄ cup, start a new jar of milk.

7. Use a sterilized spoon (rinse in boiling water if necessary, and don't use any wood utensils) to stir, then completely cover the top of your milk jar with a small sterilized dish to keep out dust, and leave the jar out at room temperature. Don't use a screw-top cap on the milk since fermenting produces some gas that needs to escape. Designate an out-of-the-way spot for your kefir; you'll be leaving it there for two to three days. Stir it once or twice during this time.

8. Start tasting the milk on the second day to determine when it's done, according to your taste preference. Again, if you won't drink it, it's not worth the process.

9. Once the kefir is ready, pour your milk through a strainer and recapture the kefir grains to use them for next time. Put the newly strained kefir grains back into a jar (don't rinse them) and place the jar in the refrigerator. Use the same jar to store your kefir grains every time, and wash it every three or four times you use it.

10. Now put your kefir milk in the refrigerator. Store your milk there for up to two weeks. It may get sour as time goes on.

Oil	Pair It With	Notes
Extra-virgin olive oil	Cold salads and vegetable dishes; use with a variety of vinegars and citrus juices such as lemon or lime juice	Use within six months of opening. Look for oil with a darker, richer color.
Olive oil, Pure or Pomace olive oil	Roasted dishes	This olive oil has a higher smoke point (over 400°F, or 200°C/ gas mark 6) than extra-virgin olive oil, so it's better to use for cooking.
Almond, Hazelnut, Macadamia, and Walnut oil	Cold salads and vegetable dishes; use with a variety of vinegars	Buy in small containers since they're expensive.
Avocado oil	Cold salads and vegetable dishes; roasted carrots or other roasted dishes	This oil has a high smoke point and can be used for both cold and cooked dishes.
Flaxseed oil	Cold salads and vegetable dishes; finish off warm dishes like wilted greens; use with a variety of vinegars	Don't cook with flaxseed oil, but since it's so healthful, feel free to top cooked dishes with the oil.
Sesame oil	Cold salads and vegetable dishes; stir-fries or roasted dishes; mix with rice vinegar and a tablespoon or two of orange juice	This oil has a high smoke point and can be used for both cold and cooked dishes.
Grapeseed oil	Cooked dishes	This flavorful oil is great for those who want to use just a little oil. This one really enhances the natural flavor of what you're cooking.
Canola oil	Cooked dishes	Lowest in saturated fat of all oils. Has heart-healthy ALAs, a precursor for omega-3 fats
Sunflower oil	Best for roasting dishes in the oven	This delicate oil has a lower smoke point but is still used for cooked dishes. Don't use this over an open flame or it will heat the oil too much.
Safflower oil	Cold salads and vegetable dishes; cooked dishes	A versatile oil that is good for both cold and cooked dishes. It won't overpower the natural taste of your foods.

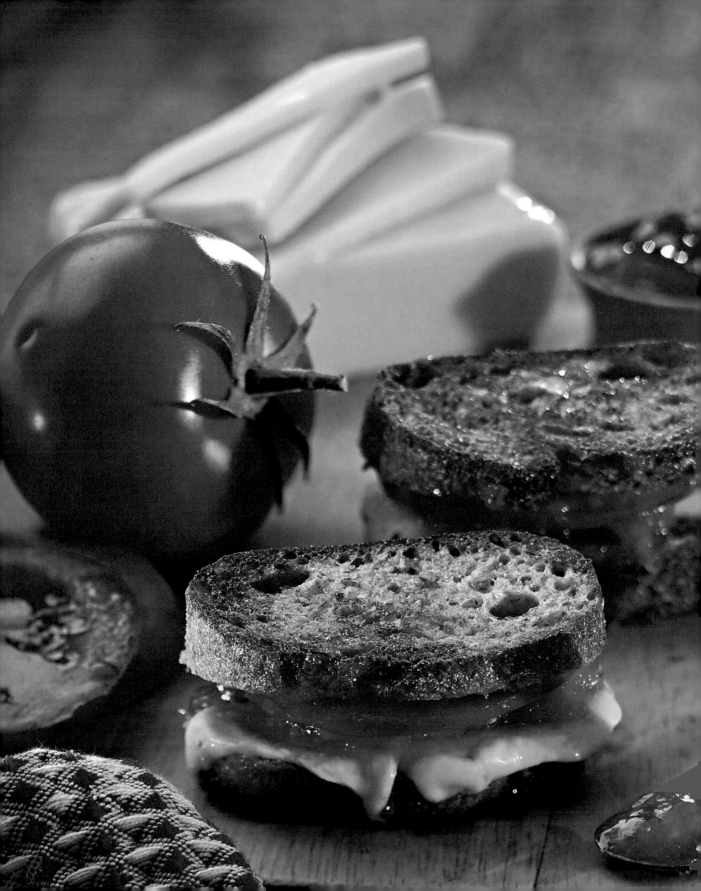

The Recipes

And now, for the easy, tasty recipes you've been waiting for. In this section, you'll find about one hundred recipes organized in four categories, including healthy breakfasts, lunches, dinners, and snacks. Some of the recipes are complete meals and some include a tip to "Make It a Meal" by adding whole grains, fruits, vegetables, or some lean protein.

When choosing yogurt, select a low-fat yogurt with the "Live & Active Cultures" seal, which means it has the probiotic starter bacteria *S. thermophilus* and *L. bulgaricus*. For any of the yogurts mentioned in the recipes, if you prefer another flavor than the one mentioned, the fruit and vanilla flavors are interchangeable with each other.

If you need to substitute an ingredient, or if there's a food you don't like, choose a food with similar nutritional content, such as a single serving of another fruit or vegetable. When berries are out of season, or if you prefer to shop less often and have berries with a longer shelf life, please choose frozen, unsweetened berries. For smoothies, try adding the berries frozen since they give the smoothie a frothy texture. Here are the single serving sizes for fruits and vegetables so you can make substitutions:

- **Fruit:** one medium-sized whole fruit, 1 cup (130 g) chopped fruit or berries, ½ cup (75 g) grapes, 2 tablespoons (30 g) dried fruit, 2 plums, 1 kiwi, or ½ cup (120 ml) fruit juice
- **Vegetables:** 1 to 2 cups (20 to 40 g) leafy vegetables, 1 cup (135 g) non-leafy vegetables, ½ cup (80 g) cooked vegetables, or ¾ cup (175 ml) low-sodium tomato juice

You may substitute or exchange any of the following within your recipes: nonfat cow's milk, 1 percent cow's milk, plain low-fat soy milk, low fat goat's milk, or low fat kofir. Smart choices to drink with your meals include tea and flavored seltzer (look for water and natural flavoring as the only ingredients).

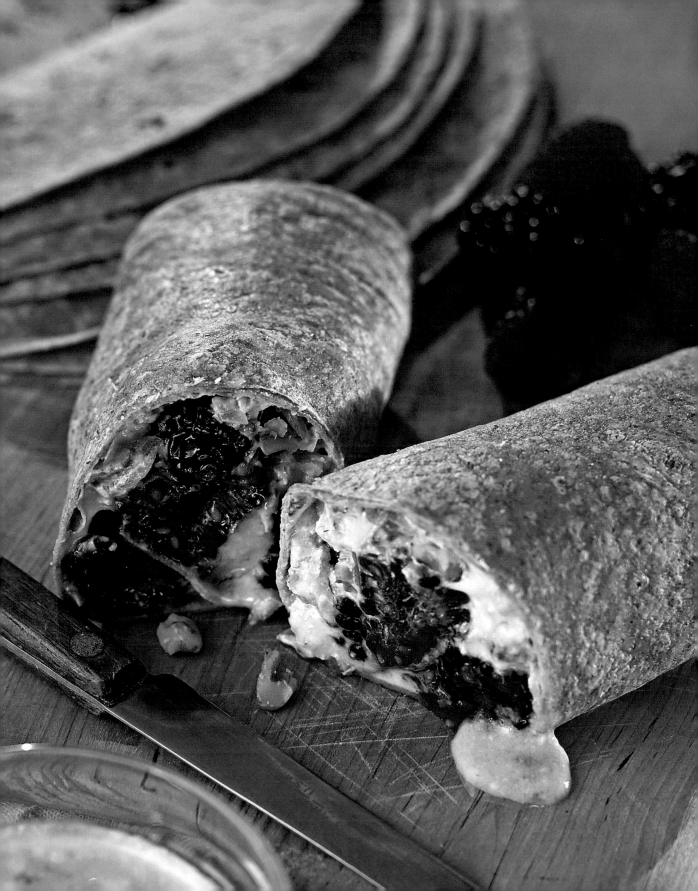

BREAKFASTS

Garden Vegetable Omelet

The heart healthy unsaturated fats in the olive oil give flavor to the veggies. The green pepper provides 100 percent of your daily value of the antioxidant vitamin C, protecting your tissues, DNA, and RNA from damage by free radicals. The colorful vegetables make this omelet mouth-watering to look at and tasty to eat!

- 2 teaspoons (10 ml) olive oil
- ½ green pepper, chopped
- ¼ cup (40 g) chopped onion
- 1 egg
- 2 egg whites or ¼ cup (60 ml) egg substitute
- ½ cup (75 g) grape tomatoes, halved

Heat a skillet over medium heat with the oil. Add the pepper and onion and sauté until onion is translucent. Whisk together egg and egg whites. Remove pepper and onion from the pan and add eggs, then sprinkle tomatoes, pepper, and onion over top of eggs. Cook until eggs are nearly set, then fold in half and continue cooking until eggs are set.

Yield: 1 serving

Each will have: 250 calories, 14 g fat, 2.9 g saturated fat, 0 g trans fat, 212 mg cholesterol, 16 g carbohydrate, 15 g protein, 184 mg sodium, 2.6 g fiber.

TIP: MAKE IT A MEAL

Serve with 1 oat bran English muffin topped with 1 teaspoon light, trans-fat-free margarine on each half.

With English muffin and margarine, each will have: 403 calories, 19 g fat, 4.2 g saturated fat, 0 g trans fat, 212 mg cholesterol, 42 g carbohydrate, 19 g protein, 450 mg sodium, 4.6 g fiber.

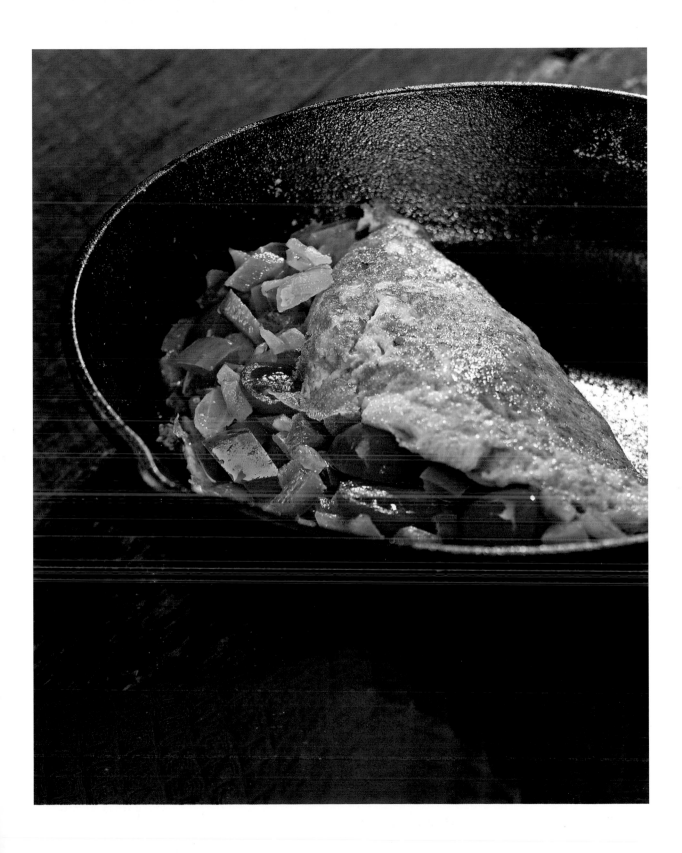

Yogurt with Honeydew

Honeydew provides soluble fiber, which feeds your probiotic bacteria, and also half of your daily requirement of vitamin C, which keeps your blood vessels healthy and aids in the absorption of iron and folate. Who says you can't have dessert for breakfast? The combination of creamy yogurt and sweet, juicy honeydew is divine.

- 4 ounces (115 g) low-fat vanilla yogurt
- 1 cup (155 g) chopped honeydew
- 2 teaspoons (5 g) ground flaxseed

In a bowl, top yogurt with honeydew and flaxseed.

Yield: 1 serving

Each will have: 198 calories, 4 g fat, 1.7 g saturated fat, 0 g trans fat, 10 mg cholesterol, 36 g carbohydrate, 7 g protein, 103 mg sodium, 2.7 g fiber.

TIP: MAKE IT A MEAL

Serve with 1 whole-grain flax bar such as Kashi TLC Granola Bar.

With Kashi TLC Pumpkin Spice Flax Granola Bar, each will have: 379 calories, 10 g fat, 2.2 g saturated fat, 0 g trans fat, 10 mg cholesterol, 62 g carbohydrate, 13 g protein, 253 mg sodium, 6.7 g fiber.

Kiwi-Strawberry Kefir Smoothie

The kiwi supplies nearly all of your daily requirement of vitamin K, and recent studies link the vitamin to increased bone density. The smoothie also packs nearly 40 percent of your calcium for the day, a surefire formula for keeping your skeleton healthy. It's the perfect mixture of sweet and sour to satisfy your morning cravings.

- 2 kiwi, peeled and diced
- 1 cup (110 g) strawberries, tops removed
- 1 cup (235 ml) low-fat kefir
- ½ teaspoon flaxseed oil
- ⅛ teaspoon pure vanilla extract

In a blender, combine all ingredients and blend until smooth.

Yield: 1 serving

Each will have: 230 calories, 5g fat, 1.8 g saturated fat, 0 g trans fat, 0 mg cholesterol, 49 g carbohydrate, 17 g protein, 131 mg sodium, 10 g fiber.

TIP: MAKE IT A MEAL

Serve with ½ cup (26 g) whole-grain, high-fiber cereal, such as Kashi Good Friends; sprinkle cereal in the smoothie and eat with a spoon.

With cereal, each will have: 300 calories, 6 g fat, 1.8 g saturated fat, 0 g trans fat, 0 mg cholesterol, 67 g carbohydrate, 19 g protein, 196 mg sodium, 16 g fiber.

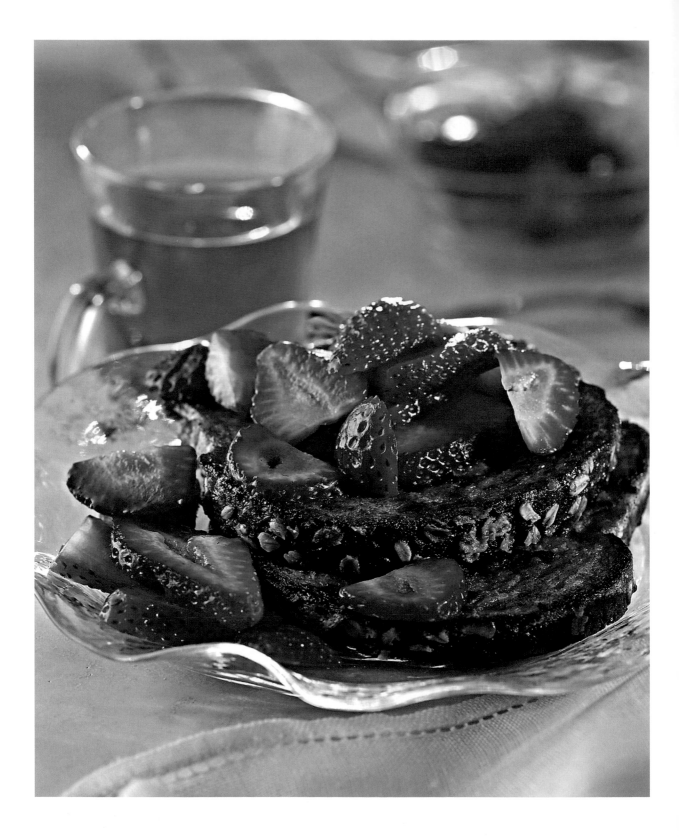

French Toast with Strawberries

This breakfast gives you a whopping nine grams of fiber, great for filling you up and helping your good digestive bacteria to flourish. Fiber also helps keep your calorie intake in check. The strawberries give you nearly three times your daily need of vitamin C.

- 1 egg
- 2 egg whites or ¼ cup (60 ml) egg substitute
- ⅓ cup (80 ml) nonfat milk
- 2 tablespoons (28 g) light, trans fat–free margarine
- 4 slices whole-wheat bread
- 2 teaspoons (10 g) brown sugar
- ¼ teaspoon ground cinnamon
- 2 cups (340 g) fresh strawberries, sliced

In a medium bowl, whisk together the eggs and milk. Melt margarine in a frying pan over medium-low heat. Dip each slice of bread into the egg mixture and add to the pan. In the pan, sprinkle bread evenly with the brown sugar and cinnamon. Turn to finish cooking on other side. Cook until eggs are set, about 5 minutes on each side. Serve 2 slices topped with 1 cup strawberries each.

Yield: 2 servings

Each will have: 335 calories, 10 g fat, 1.8 g saturated fat, 0 g trans fat, 107 mg cholesterol, 53 g carbohydrate, 17 g protein, 534 mg sodium, 9 g fiber.

TIP: MAKE IT A MEAL

Serve with 1 cup (235 ml) nonfat milk.

With milk, each will have: 418 calories, 10 g fat, 1.9 g saturated fat, 0 g trans fat, 111 mg cholesterol, 65 g carbohydrate, 25 g protein, 637 mg sodium, 9 g fiber.

Cashew English Muffin with Raspberry Smoothie

The smoothie packs over four grams of fiber, because raspberries are one of the most fiber-rich foods around! The monounsaturated fat in the cashew butter helps to keep you full until lunchtime. Choose an oat bran English muffin for a gram of soluble fiber to feed your probiotic bacteria.

For the English muffin:
- 1 oat bran English muffin
- 1 tablespoon (16 g) cashew butter

For the raspberry smoothie:
- 1 cup (235 ml) nonfat milk
- 1 teaspoon (5 ml) flaxseed oil
- ½ cup (120 ml) fresh raspberries
- ⅛ teaspoon pure almond extract

Toast the English muffin, then spread each half with half the cashew butter.

To make the smoothie, in a blender, combine the milk, flaxseed oil, raspberries, and almond extract and blend until smooth.

Yield: 1 serving

Each will have: 375 calories, 14 g fat, 2.7 g saturated fat, 0 g trans fat, 5 mg cholesterol, 51 g carbohydrate, 16 g protein, 422 mg sodium, 6.3 g fiber.

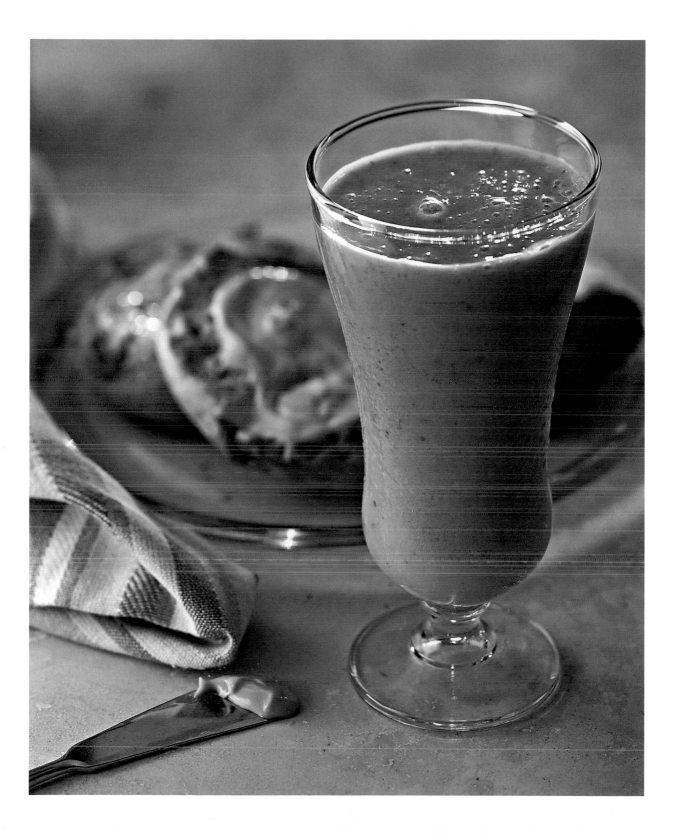

Pineapple Buttermilk Smoothie

The pineapple provides all of your daily need of manganese, an important mineral for bone health and blood sugar management. One cup of buttermilk supplies nearly a quarter of your daily requirement of phosphorus, a mineral that's essential for the formation of bones and teeth. It's a sweet and savory surprise.

- 1½ cups (233 g) fresh pineapple, chopped (or canned, packed in juice)
- 1 cup (235 ml) low-fat buttermilk
- ½ teaspoon pure vanilla extract

In a blender, combine all ingredients and blend until smooth.

Yield: 1 serving

Each will have: 216 calories, 2 g fat, 1.3 g saturated fat, 0 g trans fat, 10 mg cholesterol, 41 g carbohydrate, 9 g protein, 260 mg sodium, 3.2 g fiber.

TIP: MAKE IT A MEAL

Serve with 2 whole-wheat crackers, such as Wasa Multi Grain crispbread spread with 1 tablespoon (16 g) peanut butter (divided evenly between the 2 crackers).

With crackers and peanut butter, each will have: 400 calories, 10 g fat, 3 g saturated fat, 0 g trans fat, 10 mg cholesterol, 64 g carbohydrate, 17 g protein, 493 mg sodium, 8.2 g fiber.

Apricot Flax Oatmeal

The apricots and the milk give you 65 percent of your daily requirement of vitamin A, which helps fight infections. The soluble fiber in the apricots and the oatmeal also help maintain your good intestinal bacteria.

- ½ cup (40 g) dry oatmeal
- 1 cup (235 ml) nonfat milk
- 4 fresh apricots, sliced and pitted
- 1 tablespoon (7 g) ground flaxseed
- 1 tablespoon (8 g) pecans, chopped

Prepare oatmeal with milk. Top with apricots, flaxseed, and pecans.

Yield: 1 serving

Each will have: 385 calories, 11 g fat, 1.3 g saturated fat, 0 g trans fat, 5 mg cholesterol, 58 g carbohydrate, 17 g protein, 106 mg sodium, 9.3 g fiber.

Blueberry Cream Cereal Bowl

Blueberries are high in soluble fiber to help keep your colon functioning in top condition as well as antioxidants, which aid your body reduce cellular damage associated with aging.

- ¾ cup (169 g) low-fat fruit-flavored yogurt
- 3 tablespoons (30 g) dried blueberries
- ¾ cup (40 g) whole-grain, high-fiber cereal
- 1 tablespoon (7 g) ground flaxseed
- 1 teaspoon fresh mint

Pour yogurt into a bowl and top with blueberries, cereal, flaxseed, and mint; stir once or twice to combine.

Yield: 1 serving

Each will have: 458 calories, 6 g fat, 1.5 g saturated fat, 0 g trans fat, 7 mg cholesterol, 99 g carbohydrate, 14 g protein, 300 mg sodium, 18 g fiber.

Honey Blackberry Smoothie

The soluble fiber in the blackberries is the ideal food to fuel growth of your good bacteria. The blackberries also provide almost 40 percent of your daily need of vitamin K, also known as the "clotting vitamin" since it's essential to clot blood. Start your day off right with this sweet, purple smoothie.

- 1 cup (235 ml) low-fat kefir
- 1½ cup (195 g) fresh blackberries
- 2 teaspoons (14 g) honey
- 1 teaspoon (5 ml) flaxseed oil
- ¼ teaspoon pure vanilla extract
- ½ teaspoon fresh mint

In a blender, combine all ingredients and blend until smooth.

Yield: 1 serving

Each will have: 301 calories, 8 g fat, 2 g saturated fat, 0 g trans fat, 0 mg cholesterol, 45 g carbohydrate, 17 g protein, 138 mg sodium, 15 g fiber.

TIP: MAKE IT A MEAL

Serve with 1 slice whole-wheat toast topped with
1 tablespoon (16 g) cashew butter.

With toast and cashew butter, each will have: 475 calories, 17 g fat,
3.6 g saturated fat, 0 g trans fat, 0 mg cholesterol, 67 g carbohydrate, 24 g protein,
406 mg sodium, 18 g fiber.

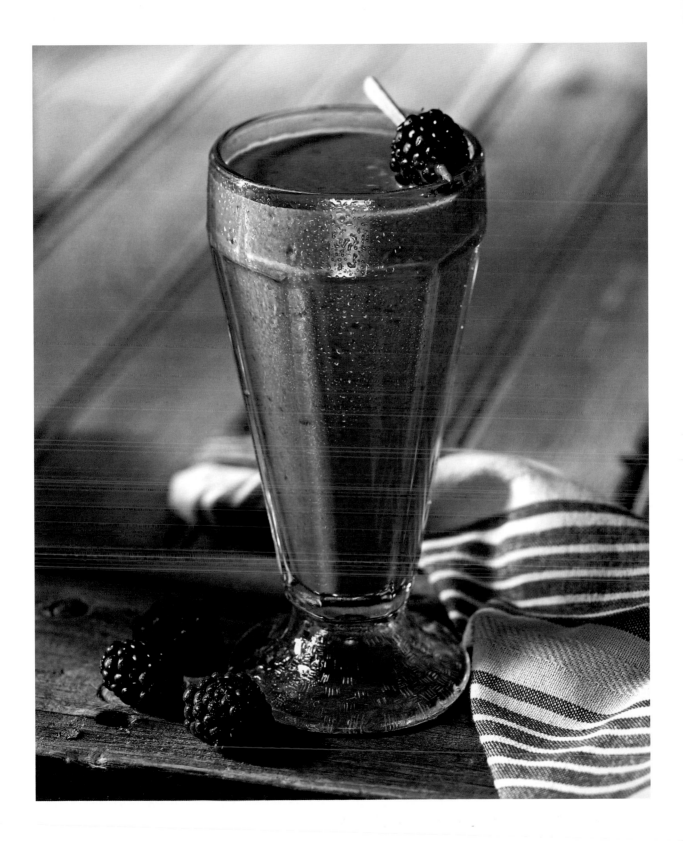

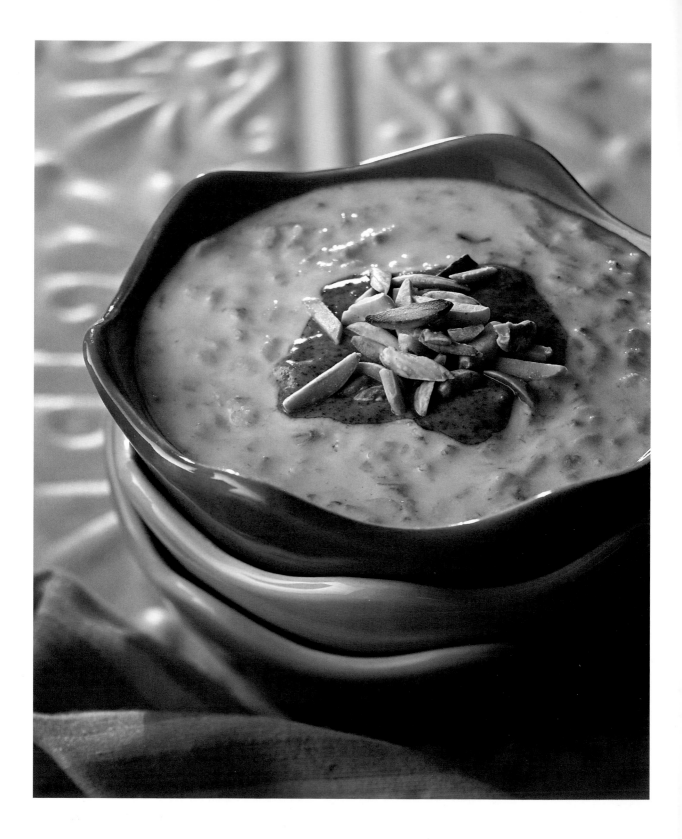

Almond Yogurt Oatmeal

The almonds and almond butter provide monounsaturated fats, which help develop and maintain your body's cells. The nutty and sweet flavors blend to make this a breakfast you'll get up early for!

- 1 tablespoon (8 g) slivered almonds
- ¾ cup (175 ml) water
- ⅓ cup (27 g) oats
- 1 tablespoon (16 g) almond butter
- 4 ounces (115 g) low-fat vanilla yogurt

Preheat oven to 250°F (120°C, or gas mark ½). Spread the almonds over a piece of aluminum foil or cookie sheet and bake for 2 minutes. Prepare oatmeal with water according to package directions. Stir in almonds, almond butter, and yogurt.

Yield: 1 serving

Each will have: 349 calories, 17 g fat, 3 g saturated fat, 0 g trans fat, 10 mg cholesterol, 42 g carbohydrate, 12 g protein, 147 mg sodium, 4 g fiber.

TIP: MAKE IT A MEAL

Serve with 1 cup (235 ml) nonfat milk.

With milk, each will have: 400 calories, 17 g fat, 3 g saturated fat, 0 g trans fat, 10 mg cholesterol, 54 g carbohydrate, 20 g protein, 250 mg sodium, 4 g fiber.

Waffles with Mango Mint Salsa

The mango provides soluble fiber, which has a positive effect on digestion from start to finish, and over 30 percent of your vitamin A requirement for the day. Vitamin A is essential for good health because it promotes growth and stability of your immune system, reproductive system, and vision. It's a minty-sweet way to start the day.

- 1 mango, chopped into small pieces
- 2½ teaspoons (15 ml) agave nectar or honey
- 1 teaspoon (2 g) fresh mint
- 2 whole-grain, high-fiber frozen waffles

Combine mango, agave nectar, and mint; toss well. Toast two waffles according to package directions and top with the mango salsa.

Yield: 1 serving

Each will have: 355 calories, 4 g fat, 0 g saturated fat, 0 g trans fat, 0 mg cholesterol, 82 g carbohydrate, 9 g protein, 335 mg sodium, 9.9 g fiber.

TIP: MAKE IT A MEAL

Serve with 4 ounces (115 g) low-fat fruit-flavored yogurt.

With yogurt, each will have: 465 calories, 6 g fat, 1 g saturated fat, 0 g trans fat, 5 mg cholesterol, 101 g carbohydrate, 14 g protein, 400 mg sodium, 9.9 g fiber.

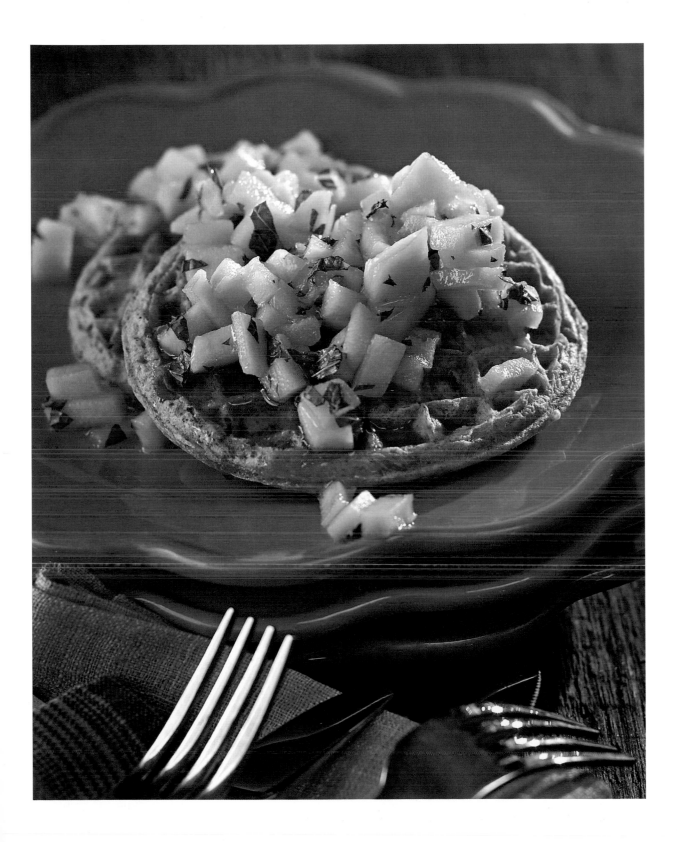

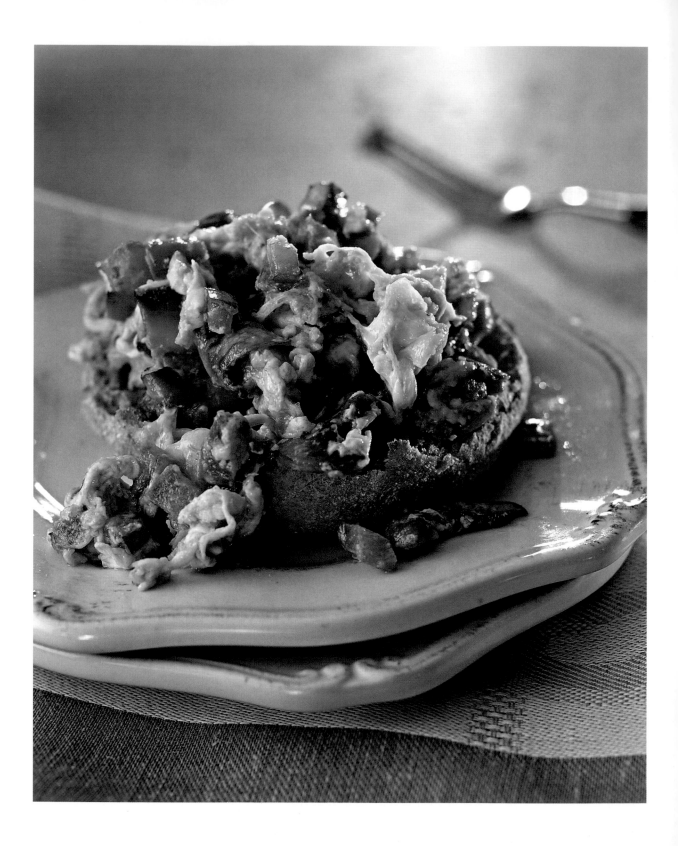

Grilled Mushroom, Pepper, and Grana Padano Scramble

The mushroom and pepper contribute fiber which helps move food and waste along in your digestive system. Eggs are sometimes called the "perfect protein" since they have all eight essential amino acids and high quality protein. In fact, eggs are the standard by which other proteins are compared! Mushrooms can sustain high temperatures in cooking and will marinate in the juices of the peppers.

- 1 teaspoon (5 ml) olive oil
- ¼ cup (18 g) white mushrooms, sliced
- ¼ cup (30 g) green pepper, chopped
- 1 egg
- 1 ounce (28 g) Grana Padano cheese, or Parmigiano-Reggiano
- 1 oat bran English muffin

Heat the olive oil in a skillet over medium-low heat. Add the mushrooms and green pepper; sauté for 4 minutes, stirring occasionally. In a small bowl, whisk the egg and add to the mushroom mixture in the skillet, stirring constantly until the egg is set, about 4 minutes. Turn off the heat and add the cheese, allowing it to melt over the mixture for 1 minute. Toast the English muffin and fill with the egg mixture.

Yield: 1 serving

Each will have: 354 calories, 19 g fat, 4.7 g saturated fat, 0 g trans fat, 212 mg cholesterol, 20 g carbohydrate, 21 g protein, 282 mg sodium, 2.9 g fiber

Tomato and Mozzarella Wrap

The cheese and tomato combine to provide over 35 percent of your daily value of vitamin A, an essential vitamin in cell differentiation, a normal process in cell development during which cells become structurally and functionally different from one another. Enjoy this delightful Mediterranean salad in a take-along version. Caprese on the go!

- 1 teaspoon (5 ml) olive oil
- 2 tomatoes, chopped
- 1 teaspoon (0.8 g) fresh thyme
- ¼ cup (30 g) shredded, part-skim mozzarella cheese
- 1 whole-grain wrap, such as Flatout Multi-Grain

Heat the olive oil in a skillet over medium-low heat. Add tomatoes and thyme and heat for 4 minutes, stirring occasionally. Turn off heat, add mozzarella, and allow cheese to melt for 1 minute. Spoon mixture into the wrap and roll up to eat.

Yield: 1 serving

Each will have: 265 calories, 14 g fat, 4 g saturated fat, 0 g trans fat, 15 mg cholesterol, 28 g carbohydrate, 24 g protein, 582 mg sodium, 11 g fiber.

TIP: MAKE IT A MEAL

Serve with 1 cup (225 g) low-fat plain yogurt topped
with 1 tablespoon (9 g) raisins.

With yogurt and raisins, each will have: 446 calories, 17 g fat, 6.6 g saturated fat,
0 g trans fat, 30 mg cholesterol, 52 g carbohydrate, 37 g protein, 754 mg sodium, 11.4 g fiber.

Crispbread with Yogurt, Flaxseed, and Blueberries

Recent research shows that flaxseeds, rich in ALA (alpha linolenic acid), can help control hot flashes in postmenopausal women. Appetizers for breakfast! Whip this sweet, creamy, crunchy combo together in just minutes.

- 4 Wasa Multi Grain crispbreads, or 1 whole-wheat soft tortilla (such as Flatout Multi-Grain) toasted and sliced into quarters
- ¾ cup (170 g) low-fat plain yogurt
- ¾ cup (109 g) blueberries
- 2 tablespoons (14 g) ground flaxseed

If using the soft tortilla, preheat the oven to 200°F (90°C, or below gas mark ½), place the tortilla on the center rack, and bake for 2 minutes. If using the Wasa crackers, skip this step. Spread the yogurt over the crackers or toasted tortilla and top with blueberries and flaxseed.

Yield: 1 serving

Each will have: 433 calories, 9 g fat, 2.4 g saturated fat, 0 g trans fat, 11 mg cholesterol, 73 g carbohydrate, 21 g protein, 454 mg sodium, 14 g fiber.

Tropical Cereal

The insoluble fiber in the cereal helps to keep stools soft and reduce your risk for diverticulosis, small pockets along the intestinal wall that can cause discomfort. The coconut has 1.5 grams of saturated fat, but coconut also has conjugated linoleic acid (CLA), which recent research has shown to be a health-promoting fatty acid. Aloha! Shredded wheat in a grass skirt.

- 1 tablespoon (5 g) shredded coconut
- 4 ounces (115 g) low-fat yogurt
- 1 cup (50 g) shredded wheat cereal
- ½ cup (78 g) fresh pineapple, cubed (or canned in juice, drained)
- 2 tablespoons (22 g) dried mango, chopped

Preheat the oven to 200°F (90°C, or below gas mark ½). Spread coconut on a piece of aluminum foil and bake for 2 minutes. Combine yogurt, cereal, pineapple, and mango, and top with the toasted coconut.

Yield: 1 serving

Each will have: 364 calories, 4 g fat, 2.6 g saturated fat, 0 g trans fat, 10 mg cholesterol, 80 g carbohydrate, 9 g protein, 75 mg sodium, 5.8 g fiber.

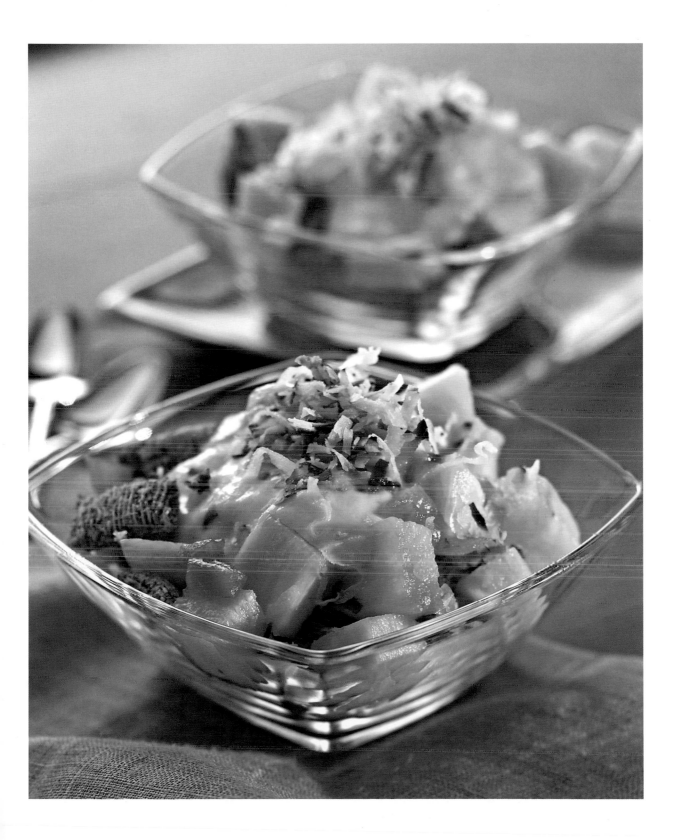

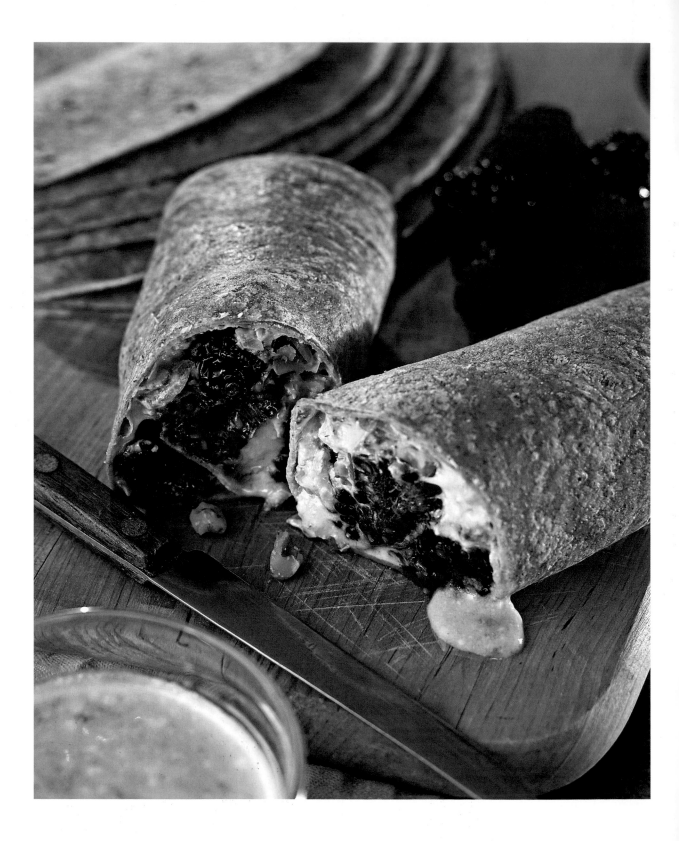

Walnut Berry Wrap

Whether you use raspberries, blackberries, blueberries, or strawberries, the phytochemicals in these "super foods" slow down tumor growth and seem to block cancer development as well as help digestion. The walnuts provide crunch and the berries make a creamy, sweet taste sensation for this simple wrap.

- 4 ounces (115 g) low-fat fruit-flavored yogurt
- 1 whole-grain wrap, such as Flatout Multi-Grain
- ½ cup (55 g) raspberries
- ½ cup (73 g) blackberries
- 2 tablespoons (16 g) walnuts, chopped

Spread the yogurt over the wrap. Fill with the raspberries, blackberries, and walnuts. Roll up to eat.

Yield: 1 serving

Each will have: 370 calories, 14 g fat, 1.5 g saturated fat, 0 g trans fat, 10 mg cholesterol, 52 g carbohydrate, 19 g protein, 452 mg sodium, 17 g fiber.

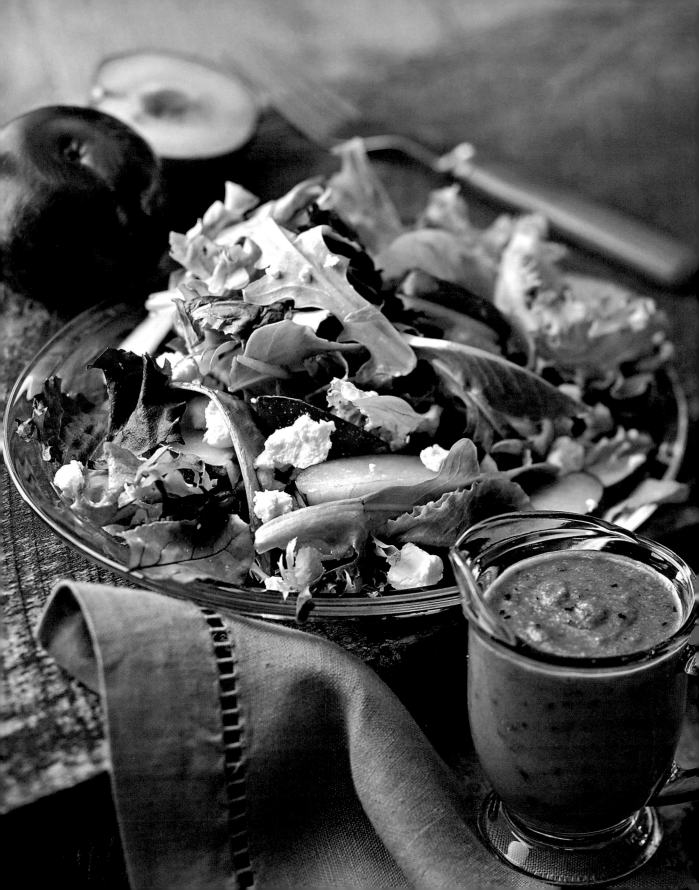

LUNCHES

Tempeh Cubes with Ginger Vegetables

Tempeh is a soy product that's rich in probiotic bacteria. It's made from the versatile soybean, which supplies all eight of the essential amino acids, making it a great source of protein. The distinctive ginger taste is sure to make this recipe a new favorite.

- 1 cup (235 ml) water
- ½ cup (80 g) tempeh
- 1 tablespoon (14 g) light, trans-fat-free margarine
- 1 egg
- ½ cup (35 g) broccoli florets
- 2 scallions, chopped
- 1 teaspoon minced ginger
- 1 teaspoon minced garlic

In a small saucepan over medium-low heat, simmer the water and the tempeh for 10 minutes. Remove from heat, place tempeh on several paper towels to drain; when dry, cut tempeh into cubes.

Melt margarine in a skillet over medium-low heat; add tempeh and sauté, stirring occasionally for 4 minutes. Add egg, broccoli, scallions, garlic, and ginger and continue to sauté, stirring occasionally, for another 5 minutes.

Yield: 1 serving

Each will have: 324 calories, 19 g fat, 4.4 g saturated fat, 0 g trans fat, 212 mg cholesterol, 9 g carbohydrate, 25 g protein, 198 mg sodium, 3.2 g fiber.

TIP: MAKE IT A MEAL

Serve over ½ cup (82 g) cooked brown rice.

With rice, each will have: 433 calories, 20 g fat, 4.6 g saturated fat, 0 g trans fat, 212 mg cholesterol, 40 g carbohydrate, 27 g protein, 199 mg sodium, 5 g fiber.

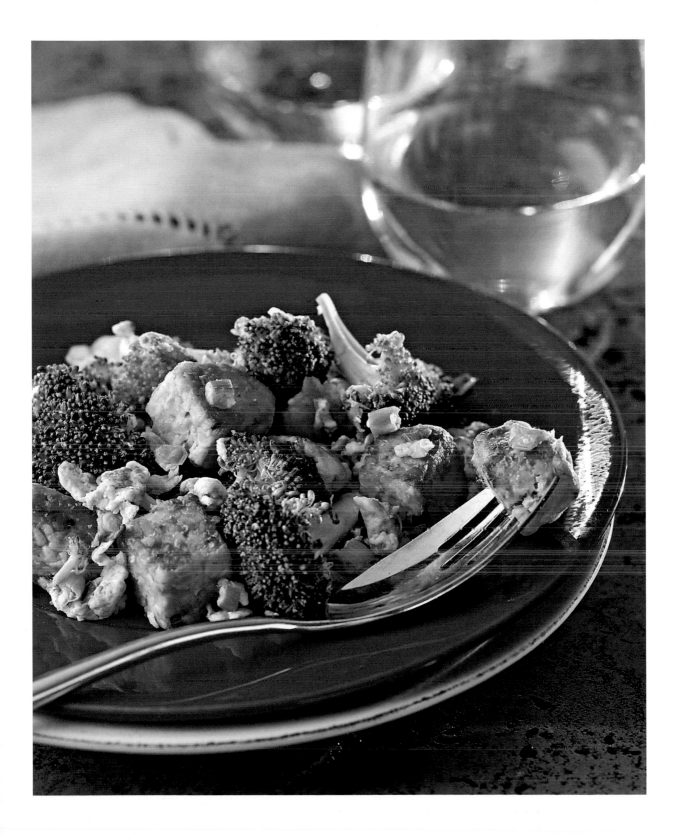

Super Kefir Smoothie

This kefir-based smoothie is one of the few drinks you can find that provides fiber. One cup has 3 grams of fiber, which helps you feel full faster, improves your digestion and can help control your weight. This is truly a meal in a glass! Enjoy for a complete lunch on the run.

- 1 cup (235 ml) low-fat kefir
- 1 cup (140 g) frozen, unsweetened blackberries
- 2 teaspoons (10 ml) flaxseed oil
- 4 ounces (115 g) low-fat fruit-flavored yogurt
- ¼ cup (60 ml) orange juice
- ¼ cup (60 ml) pomegranate juice
- 2 ounces (60 g) firm, silken tofu
- ½ teaspoon pure vanilla extract

Combine all ingredients in a blender and blend until smooth.

Yield: 1 serving

Each will have: 442 calories, 9 g fat, 3 g saturated fat, 0 g trans fat, 5 mg cholesterol, 66 g carbohydrate, 26 g protein, 267 mg sodium, 11 g fiber.

TIP: MAKE IT A MEAL

Serve with 2 cups (40 g) mixed baby greens topped
with 1 tablespoon (15 ml) balsamic vinegar.

With greens and balsamic vinegar, each will have: 477 calories, 9 g fat, 3 g saturated fat, 0 g trans fat, 5 mg cholesterol, 72 g carbohydrate, 27 g protein, 298 mg sodium, 12 g fiber.

Navy Bean Spread

These small white beans are a good source of cholesterol-lowering fiber and folate, a vitamin that reduces the risk of stroke. The fiber is also proven to lower women's risk for gallstones, since it lowers the level of cholesterol in bile and reduces the chance for gallstone formation. Roasted garlic lends a subtle flavor to this filling spread.

- 3 cloves garlic
- 1 cup (225 g) navy beans, soaked and drained or canned, rinsed and drained
- 1 teaspoon olive oil
- 1 tablespoon (15 ml) water
- 1/16 teaspoon salt
- 1/4 teaspoon ground black pepper
- 1/2 teaspoon fresh rosemary
- 1 whole-wheat soft tortilla, such as Flatout Multi-Grain

Preheat the oven to 400°F (200°C, or gas mark 6). Wrap garlic in foil and place directly on the middle rack in the oven to bake for 20 minutes. This can be done up to three days in advance; store roasted garlic in a resealable plastic bag at room temperature. Turn heat down to 220°F (90°C, or gas mark 1/2) and place tortilla on center rack and bake for 2 minutes. Break tortilla into triangles.

In a blender, combine garlic, navy beans, olive oil, water, salt, pepper, and rosemary, and use the pulse action to blend the ingredients until well blended. Dip the bean spread with the tortilla triangles.

Yield: 1 serving

Each will have: 494 calories, 9 g fat, 0.8 g saturated fat, 0 g trans fat, 0 mg cholesterol, 84 g carbohydrate, 29 g protein, 532 mg sodium, 24 g fiber.

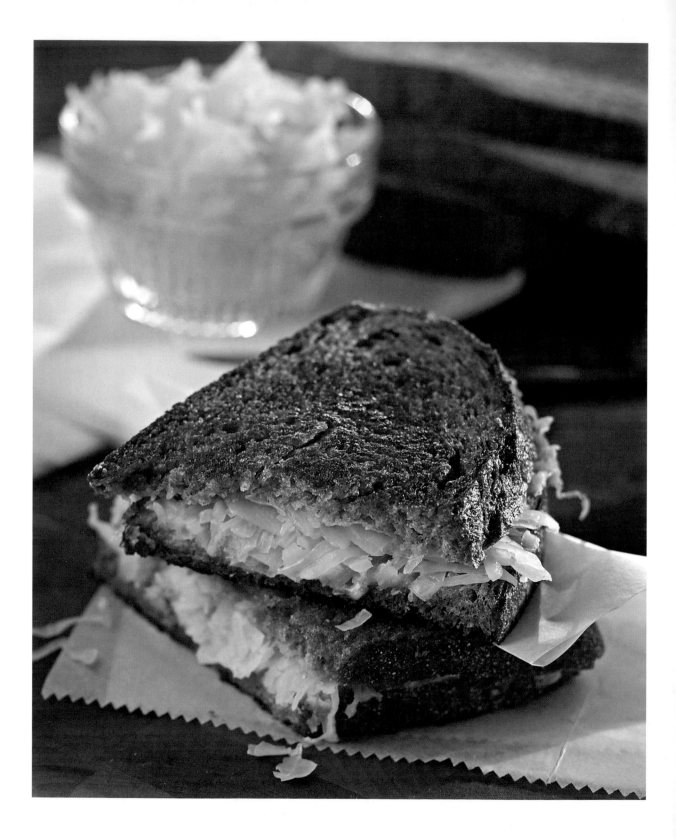

Grilled Gruyère Sandwich with Sauerkraut

The flavors in this sandwich blend together to make a tangy, tasty dish. Sauerkraut aids the absorption of iron from foods. Iron is an essential mineral that helps deliver oxygen to cells. This one is unusual, but worth trying!

- 2 slices whole-wheat bread
- 1½ tablespoons (21 g) light, trans-fat-free margarine
- 1 ounce (28 g) Gruyère cheese, or fontina, sliced
- ⅓ cup (75 g) canned sauerkraut, drained

Preheat a skillet over medium heat. Spread half of the margarine on 1 side of one slice of bread; place bread margarine-side down in the pan. Top bread with cheese and sauerkraut. Spread remaining margarine on one side of the second slice of bread; place bread margarine-side up on top of sauerkraut. Heat until cheese begins to melt, about 4 minutes. Flip sandwich and cook the other side for 3 to 4 minutes. Slice sandwich in half to eat.

Yield: 1 serving

Each will have: 352 calories, 19 g fat, 6.9 g saturated fat, 0 g trans fat, 31 mg cholesterol, 36 g carbohydrate, 16 g protein, 1037 mg sodium, 7.3 g fiber.

TIP: MAKE IT A MEAL

Serve with 1 cup (150 g) red grapes.

With grapes, each will have: 456 calories, 19 g fat, 6.9 g saturated fat, 0 g trans fat, 31 mg cholesterol, 63 g carbohydrate, 18 g protein, 1041 mg sodium, 8.7 g fiber.

Stir-Fried Chinese Vegetables

Broccoli contains insoluble fiber to aid digestion as well as phytonutrients and folate. Phytonutrients may help control diabetes and heart disease, and folate is a vitamin that aids in the production and maintenance of new cell development, which is essential for growth during childhood and pregnancy. Genuine Chinese vegetables offer a crispy crunch at mealtime.

- 2 teaspoons (10 ml) sesame oil
- ½ cup (60 g) leeks, chopped
- ½ cup (100 g) water chestnuts
- ½ cup (35 g) broccoli florets
- ½ cup (65 g) carrots, sliced
- 1 teaspoon (5 ml) reduced-sodium soy sauce
- 2 tablespoons (30 ml) rice vinegar
- 1 tablespoon (8 g) sesame seeds

Heat the oil in a skillet over medium heat. Add the leeks, water chestnuts, broccoli, and carrots and sauté for 5 minutes. Add soy sauce, rice vinegar, and sesame seeds and stir constantly for about 3 minutes.

Yield: 1 serving

Each will have: 237 calories, 14 g fat, 2 g saturated fat, 0 g trans fat, 0 mg cholesterol, 23 g carbohydrate, 5 g protein, 265 mg sodium, 5.7 g fiber.

TIP: MAKE IT A MEAL

Serve over ¾ cup (124 g) cooked brown rice.

With brown rice, each will have: 401 calories, 15 g fat, 2.2 g saturated fat, 0 g trans fat, 0 mg cholesterol, 58 g carbohydrate, 8 g protein, 267 mg sodium, 8.4 g fiber.

Dandelion Greens

Dandelion greens, a member of the sunflower family, support digestion and reduce inflammation. A tart, tangy side dish to pair nicely with any meal.

- 2 cups (40 g) dandelion greens
- 1 tablespoon (14 g) light, trans fat–free margarine
- 1 tablespoon (4 g) fresh parsley, chopped
- ⅛ teaspoon salt
- ¼ teaspoon ground black pepper
- ½ teaspoon garlic, minced
- 1 teaspoon pimento

Soak dandelion greens in water for 1 hour (this can be done in advance; store the greens in the refrigerator for up to three days wrapped in paper towels and stored in a resealable plastic bag). Rinse well and pat dry.

Melt margarine in a skillet over medium heat and add greens; sauté for 4 minutes, stirring occasionally. Reduce heat to medium-low, then add parsley, salt, pepper, garlic, and pimento and sauté for another 5 minutes, stirring occasionally.

Yield: 1 serving

Each will have: 105 calories, 5.8 g fat, 1.2 g saturated fat, 0 g trans fat, 0 mg cholesterol, 11 g carbohydrate, 3 g protein, 316 mg sodium, 4.2 g fiber

---

TIP: MAKE IT A MEAL

Serve with 1 egg and 2 egg whites scrambled in 1 teaspoon (5 ml) canola oil and 2 whole-wheat crackers, such as Wasa Multi Grain crispbread, each spread with 1 teaspoon (5 g) tahini, and half a sliced red pear.

With eggs, crackers, tahini, and pear, each will have: 439 calories, 16 g fat, 3.5 g saturated fat, 0 g trans fat, 212 mg cholesterol, 60 g carbohydrate, 20 g protein, 606 mg sodium, 13.8 g fiber.

Cabbage Wrap

Cabbage greens and shredded carrots are now available bagged and ready to use. Cabbage is a cruciferous vegetable rich in phytochemicals which help reduce the risk of colorectal cancer. Lime juice and almonds add zest to this easy wrap.

- 2 tablespoons (16 g) slivered almonds
- ½ cup (45 g) chopped red cabbage
- ½ cup (45 g) chopped green cabbage
- ¼ cup (30 g) grated carrots
- 1 tablespoon (10 g) chopped red onion
- 1 tablespoon (14 g) light canola oil mayonnaise
- 2 teaspoons (10 ml) lime juice
- 1 whole-grain wrap, such as Flatout Multi-Grain

Preheat the oven to 250°F (120°C, or gas mark ½). Spread the almonds over a piece of aluminum foil or cookie sheet and bake for 2 minutes. In a bowl, combine cabbage, carrots, onion, mayonnaise, lime juice, and almonds and stir to combine. Spoon mixture onto the wrap and roll up to eat.

Yield: 1 wrap

Each will have: 260 calories, 14 g fat, 1 g saturated fat, 0 g trans fat, 5 mg cholesterol, 30 g carbohydrate, 13 g protein, 505 mg sodium, 12 g fiber.

TIP: MAKE IT A MEAL

Serve with 4 ounces (115 g) low-fat fruit-flavored yogurt

topped with ½ cup (75 g) grapes.

With yogurt and grapes, each will have: 422 calories, 16 g fat, 2 g saturated fat, 0 g trans fat, 10 mg cholesterol, 63 g carbohydrate, 18 g protein, 572 mg sodium, 12.8 g fiber.

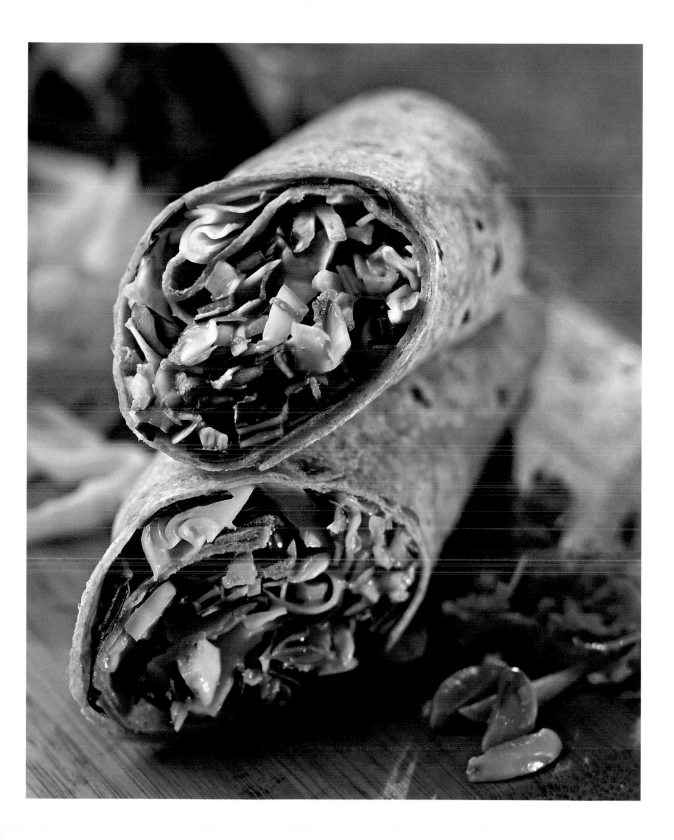

Agave Dip

Jicama, also known as yam bean or Mexican turnip, provides 25 percent of your daily requirement of vitamin C, and the fiber in this root vegetable speeds food through the digestive system. A dip tailor-made for your sweet tooth, it's great for dipping anything from vegetables to crackers.

- 4 ounces (115 g) low-fat vanilla yogurt
- 4 ounces (115 g) low-fat plain yogurt
- 1½ teaspoons agave nectar or honey
- ⅛ teaspoon ground cinnamon
- 1/16 teaspoon salt
- 1 cup (130 g) cubed jicama
- 10 baby carrots
- 2 whole-wheat crackers, such as Wasa Multi Grain crispbread

Using a wire whisk, whisk together yogurt, agave nectar, cinnamon, and salt until smooth. If preferred, you can use a food processor instead of whisking. Dip vegetables and crackers.

Yield: 1 serving

Each will have: 386 calories, 4 g fat, 2.7 g saturated fat, 0 g trans fat, 17 mg cholesterol, 76 g carbohydrate, 17 g protein, 537 mg sodium, 13 g fiber.

TIP: MAKE IT A MEAL

Serve with 1 cup (20 g) mixed baby greens topped with ½ cup (35 g) broccolini and dressed with 1 tablespoon (15 ml) balsamic vinegar.

With salad, each will have: 414 calories, 4 g fat, 2.7 g saturated fat, 0 g trans fat, 17 mg cholesterol, 81 g carbohydrate, 18 g protein, 559 mg sodium, 15 g fiber.

Artichoke and White Bean Dip

A vegetable native to the Mediterranean region, artichokes are low in calories and rich in potassium, a mineral that helps regulate the activity of muscle tissue, including the muscles of the heart and skeletal muscles.

For the dip:

- 1 (16-ounce, or 450-g) can white beans, rinsed and drained
- 6 canned artichoke hearts, drained
- 1 clove garlic, minced
- 2 tablespoons (30 ml) lemon juice
- ¼ teaspoon salt
- 2 teaspoons (10 ml) olive oil

Serve with:

- 2 tomatoes, chopped
- 4 (6-inch, or 15-cm) whole-wheat pitas

To make the dip, purée the beans, artichoke hearts, garlic, lemon juice, and salt in a food processor or blender until smooth. With the machine running, slowly add the olive oil until it is completely incorporated. To assemble, fill each pita with one quarter of the mixture and one half chopped tomato.

Yield: 4 servings

Each will have: 276 calories, 4 g fat, 0.0 g saturated fat, 0 g trans fat, 0 mg cholesterol, 55 g carbohydrate, 15 g protein, 753 mg sodium, 11 g fiber.

TIP: MAKE IT A MEAL

Serve with 2 cups (40 g) baby spinach greens topped
with ½ cup (85 g) strawberries and 1 tablespoon (9 g) pine nuts and dress
with 1 tablespoon (15 ml) balsamic vinegar.

With spinach salad, each will have: 390 calories, 11 g fat, 1 g saturated fat, 0 g trans
fat, 17 mg cholesterol, 68 g carbohydrate, 18 g protein, 804 mg sodium, 14 g fiber.

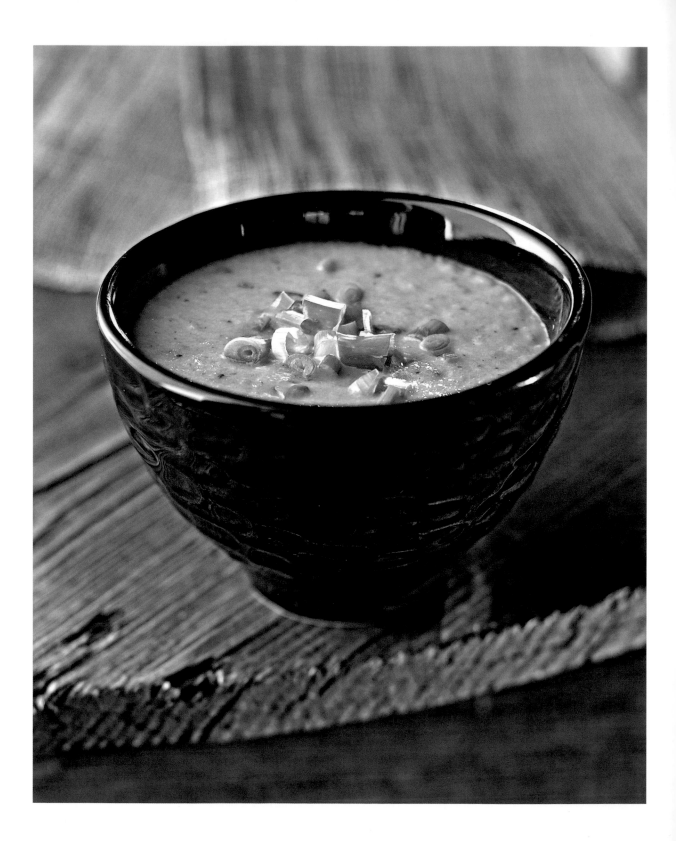

Yellow Squash and Basil Soup

Yellow squash is a source of copper, a mineral important to the health of connective tissues, including muscle and nerve tissues. Who says you can't have soup in the summer?

- 2 teaspoons (10 ml) grapeseed oil
- 1 white onion, chopped
- 1 clove garlic, minced
- 4 medium yellow summer squash, cut into ¼-inch (0.5-cm) slices
- 1 teaspoon (1 g) fresh sage, chopped
- 2 teaspoons (2 g) fresh basil, chopped
- ½ teaspoon salt
- 2 cups (475 ml) nonfat milk
- ¼ teaspoon ground black pepper
- 2 teaspoons (4 g) chopped scallions, optional

Heat the grapeseed oil in a saucepan over medium-low heat. Add the onion and garlic and sauté for 5 minutes. Add the squash, sage, basil, and salt; stir, cover, and continue to cook for another 7 minutes. Remove from heat and purée the squash mixture with the milk and pepper. Divide soup between two bowls and top each with 1 teaspoon (2 g) chopped scallions, if desired.

Yield: 2 (2½-cup, or 570-ml) servings

Each will have: 190 calories, 6 g fat, 0.7 g saturated fat, 0 g trans fat, 5 mg cholesterol, 26 g carbohydrate, 11 g protein, 404 mg sodium, 5 g fiber

---

TIP: MAKE IT A MEAL

Serve with 4 whole-wheat crackers topped with 1 tablespoon (14 g) each black bean dip and 1 serving of fruit (such as a sliced green apple).

With crackers and bean dip, each will have: 502 calories, 6 g fat, 0.7 g saturated fat, 0 g trans fat, 5 mg cholesterol, 95 g carbohydrate, 27 g protein, 955 mg sodium, 20 g fiber.

Hummus, Garbanzo Bean, and Vegetable Wrap

Garbanzo beans, or chickpeas, are a legume rich in cholesterol-lowering fiber. So if you're tired of the same old lunch, add some excitement at mealtime with this wrap.

- 1 whole-grain wrap, such as Flatout Multi-Grain
- ¼ cup (56 g) hummus
- 1 teaspoon chopped fresh basil
- 1 teaspoon lemon juice
- ¼ cup (60 g) garbanzo beans
- 1 cup (150 g) grape or cherry tomatoes, halved

Spread wrap with hummus. In a small bowl, combine basil, lemon juice, garbanzo beans, and cherry tomatoes. Spoon mixture into wrap and roll up.

Yield: 1 serving

Each will have: 294 calories, 9 g fat, 0.1 g saturated fat, 0 g trans fat, 0 mg cholesterol, 46 g carbohydrate, 15 g protein, 744 mg sodium, 13 g fiber.

TIP: MAKE IT A MEAL

Serve with 1 cup (145 g) blueberries and 1 cup (235 ml) nonfat milk.

With blueberries and milk, each will have: 460 calories, 10 g fat, 0.3 g saturated fat, 0 g trans fat, 5 mg cholesterol, 79 g carbohydrate, 24 g protein, 744 mg sodium, 17 g fiber.

Baked Potato with Sauerkraut

Just the kick you've been searching for to dress up your plain baked potato. For variety, substitute ½ cup (112 g) of probiotic-rich kimchi for the sauerkraut. Potatoes are one of the richest sources of potassium, an electrolyte that plays an essential role in nerve stimulation and muscle contraction.

- 1 large (6-ounce, or 180-g) potato
- 2 tablespoons (15 g) light sour cream
- ½ cup (112 g) canned sauerkraut
- ½ teaspoon fresh dill weed
- ½ teaspoon ground black pepper

Preheat the oven to 375°F (190°C, or gas mark 5). Pierce the potato with a fork at 1-inch (2.5-cm) intervals, wrap in aluminum foil, and place directly on middle rack in the oven; bake for 45 minutes. Allow the potato to cool, then top with sour cream, sauerkraut, and dill.

Yield: 1 serving

Each will have: 194 calories, 3 g fat, 1.7 g saturated fat, 0 g trans fat, 8 mg cholesterol, 37 g carbohydrate, 5 g protein, 755 mg sodium, 5.7 g fiber.

TIP: MAKE IT A MEAL

Serve with 1 cup (240 g) garbanzo beans, rinsed and drained, mixed with 1 teaspoon (5 ml) olive oil, 1 teaspoon (5 ml) white vinegar, ½ teaspoon (0.5 g) chopped fresh basil, and 10 halved grape tomatoes.

With garbanzo bean salad, each will have: 554 calories, 10 g fat, 2.6 g saturated fat, 0 g trans fat, 8 mg cholesterol, 99 g carbohydrate, 17 g protein, 1390 mg sodium, 17 g fiber.

Spicy Tofu Sandwich

The whole grain bread provides fiber as well as magnesium, folate, and vitamin E. Magnesium is a mineral your muscles and nerves use to relax, an important step in muscle and nerve function. Tofu can be flavorful! The mustard and parsley combine to give this sandwich a kick.

- 3 ounces (90 g) firm tofu, chopped into small chunks
- 2 teaspoons (10 g) Dijon mustard
- 1/16 teaspoon salt
- 1/8 teaspoon ground black pepper
- 1 tablespoon (8 g) grated carrots
- 1 tablespoon (6 g) chopped celery
- 2 tablespoons (28 g) low-fat plain yogurt
- 1 teaspoon flaxseed oil
- 2 teaspoons (2.6 g) parsley, chopped
- 2 slices whole-wheat bread

In a bowl, lightly toss tofu, mustard, salt, pepper, carrots, celery, yogurt, flaxseed oil, and parsley. Spoon mixture between the slices of bread.

Yield: 1 serving

Each will have: 294 calories, 10 g fat, 1.5 g saturated fat, 0 g trans fat, 2 mg cholesterol, 41 g carbohydrate, 17 g protein, 687 mg sodium, 7.2 g fiber.

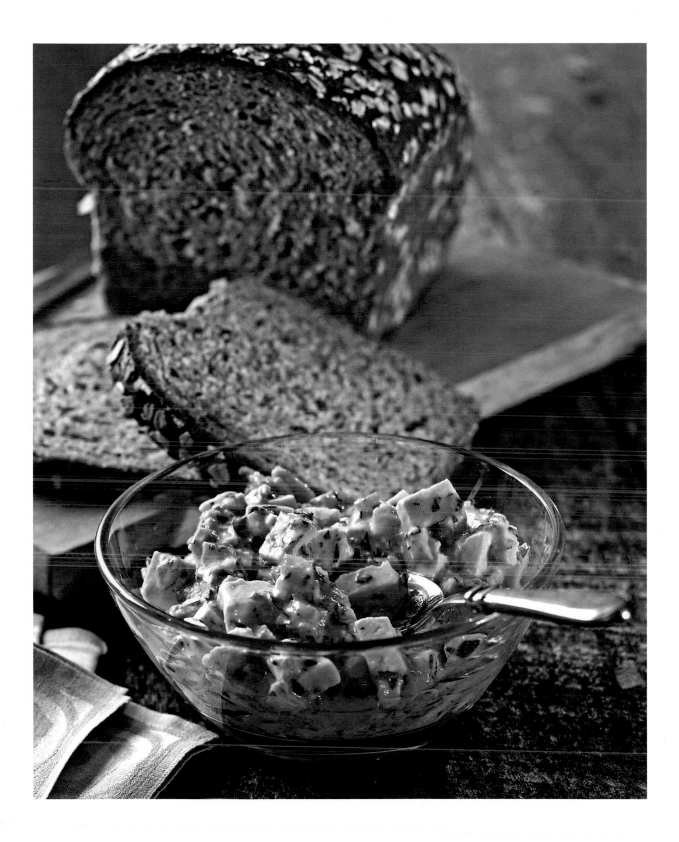

Collard Greens with Balsamic Vinegar

This superstar vegetable is from the brassica *genus of foods. A cup of collard greens provides 1.5 grams of fiber to improve digestion as well as more than 100 percent of your needs of vitamin K and vitamin A, and more than 50 percent of your daily requirement of vitamin C and manganese.*

- 1 teaspoon olive oil
- 1½ cups (30 g) collard greens
- ¹⁄₁₆ teaspoon salt
- ⅛ teaspoon ground black pepper
- 1 teaspoon balsamic vinegar
- 2 teaspoons (5 g) ground flaxseed

Heat the olive oil in a skillet over medium heat. Add collard greens to the pan and season with salt and pepper. Toss until wilted, about 2 minutes. Add balsamic vinegar and cook for another 2 minutes, tossing constantly. Remove from heat; stir in ground flaxseed.

Yield: 1 serving

Each will have: 85 calories, 7 g fat, 0.8 g saturated fat, 0 g trans fat, 30 mg cholesterol, 5 g carbohydrate, 2 g protein, 133 mg sodium, 3.3 g fiber.

TIP: MAKE IT A MEAL

Serve with 1 cup (225 g) low-fat plain yogurt topped with 2 tablespoons (16 g) chopped walnuts and 2 whole-wheat crackers, such as Wasa Multi Grain crispbread.

With yogurt, walnuts, and crackers, each will have: 426 calories, 20 g fat, 3.8 g saturated fat, 0 g trans fat, 15 mg cholesterol, 44 g carbohydrate, 22 g protein, 488 mg sodium, 8.4 g fiber.

Spinach Salad with Lemon Lentils

Lentils are legumes that are an excellent source of soluble fiber, molybdenum, and folate. The mineral molybdenum is involved in protein synthesis, an important process since proteins are hard at work in your body all day long, digesting food and transmitting nerve signals. The lemon gives a hint of flavor to the lentils, making this the perfect light lunch.

- ½ cup (225 g) lentils canned, such as Westbrae Natural Organic Lentils
- 2 teaspoons (2.6 g) parsley, chopped
- 1½ teaspoons olive oil, divided
- 1 tablespoon (15 ml) lemon juice
- ¹⁄₁₆ teaspoon salt
- 3 cups (60 g) baby spinach greens
- 1 (6-inch, or 15-cm) whole-wheat pita bread
- ⅛ teaspoon garlic powder

In a bowl, combine lentils with parsley, 1 teaspoon (5 ml) olive oil, lemon juice, and salt. Stir in the spinach greens. Preheat the oven to 200°F (90°C, or below gas mark ½).

Open and drizzle pita with remaining olive oil and sprinkle with garlic powder. Bake on the center rack of the oven for 2 minutes. Break pita into small pieces and sprinkle over the salad.

Yield: 1 serving

Each will have: 393 calories, 10 g fat, 1.3 g saturated fat, 0 g trans fat, 0 mg cholesterol, 62 g carbohydrate, 18 g protein, 559 mg sodium, 11 g fiber.

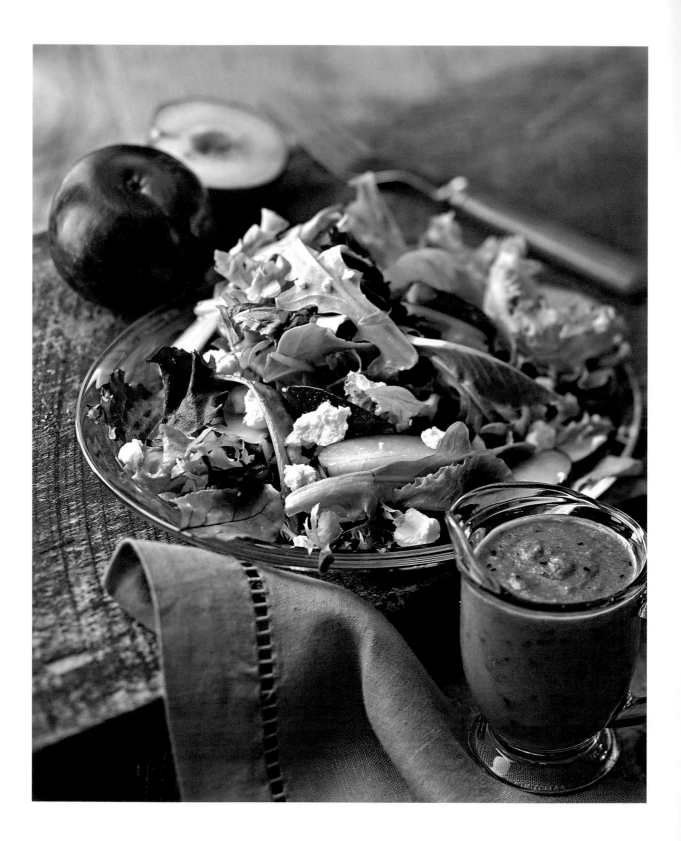

Balsamic Plum Salad

One plum provides one gram of soluble fiber, which is helpful to lower bad or LDL cholesterol. The soluble fiber decreases the reabsorption of cholesterol from foods as they travel through your digestive system. The plum is puréed and the balsamic vinegar helps bring out the flavor.

For the dressing:

- 3 plums, sliced and pitted, divided
- 1 tablespoon (10 g) chopped onion
- 1½ tablespoons (23 ml) white vinegar
- 1 tablespoon (15 ml) balsamic vinegar
- ½ teaspoon minced garlic
- 1 teaspoon olive oil
- 1/16 teaspoon salt
- 1/8 teaspoon ground black pepper

For the salad:

- 2 tablespoons (5 g) basil, chopped
- 3 cups (60 g) mixed greens
- 2 ounces (60 g) soft goat cheese, broken into small pieces
- 1 cup (30 g) whole-wheat croutons, optional

To make the dressing, use a food processor to purée 1 plum, onion, white vinegar, balsamic vinegar, garlic, olive oil, salt, and pepper.

To assemble the salad, in a large bowl, combine the basil and mixed greens; top with goat cheese, remaining plums, croutons, and the dressing.

Yield: 1 serving

Each will have: 419 calories, 19 g fat, 9 g saturated fat, 0 g trans fat, 26 mg cholesterol, 46 g carbohydrate, 17 g protein, 569 mg sodium, 6.4 g fiber.

Lime Cod Salad

Cod is a great source of selenium, which helps control damage to blood vessels in your body from oxidative stress. You get 60 percent of your daily need of selenium from this dish. And, in just minutes, you can have this citrus-flavored fish ready to serve.

- Olive oil–flavored cooking spray
- 4 ounces (115 g) cod
- 2 teaspoons (2g) fresh dill
- 2 cups (40 g) arugula greens
- 1 tablespoon (15 ml) lime juice
- 1 teaspoon (5 ml) avocado oil, or olive oil
- 1 tablespoon (1 g) cilantro, chopped
- ⅛ teaspoon salt

Preheat oven to 375°F (190°C, or gas mark 5). Sprinkle fish with fresh dill. Spray fish and baking sheet with cooking spray; place fish on prepared baking sheet. Cook about 6 minutes or until fish looks translucent and just starts to flake apart.

Dress arugula with lime juice, oil, cilantro, and salt. Flake fish over the salad.

Yield: 1 serving

Each will have: 149 calories, 6 g fat, 1 g saturated fat, 0 g trans fat, 49 mg cholesterol, 3 g carbohydrate, 21 g protein, 364 mg sodium, 0.7 g fiber.

TIP: MAKE IT A MEAL

Serve with 1 large baked sweet potato topped with 2 tablespoons (28 g) low-fat plain yogurt mixed with a drop of vanilla extract.

With sweet potato, yogurt, and vanilla extract, each will have: 386 calories, 6 g fat, 1.2 g saturated fat, 0 g trans fat, 51 mg cholesterol, 56 g carbohydrate, 27 g protein, 525 mg sodium, 8.4 g fiber.

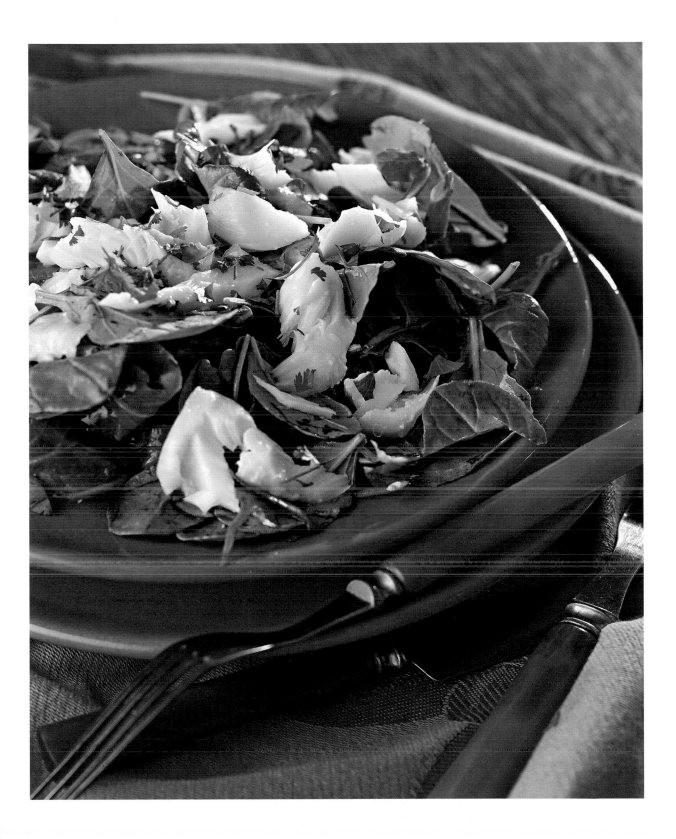

Carrots, Pear, and Pecan Salad

This dish provides more than one third of your daily requirement of chromium, a mineral that plays an active role in the glucose tolerance factor, which helps to manage your blood-sugar levels.

<u>For the dressing:</u>
- 2 tablespoons (28 g) low-fat plain yogurt
- 1 tablespoon (14 g) light canola oil mayonnaise
- 1 teaspoon sherry vinegar
- ⅟₁₆ teaspoon salt

<u>For the salad:</u>
- 1 cup (120 g) grated carrot
- 1 green pear, finely chopped
- 1 tablespoon (8 g) pecans, chopped

To make the dressing, in a small bowl whisk together the yogurt, mayonnaise, vinegar, and salt.

To assemble the salad, in a large bowl combine the carrots, pear, and pecans; toss with the dressing.

Yield: 1 serving

Each will have: 256 calories, 11 g fat, 1.6 g saturated fat, 0 g trans fat, 7 mg cholesterol, 41 g carbohydrate, 4 g protein, 344 mg sodium, 8.9 g fiber.

TIP: MAKE IT A MEAL

Serve with 1 cup (235 ml) low-fat kefir and 4 whole-wheat crackers, such as Wasa Multi Grain crispbread.

With kefir and crackers, each will have: 466 calories, 13 g fat, 3 g saturated fat, 0 g trans fat, 7 mg cholesterol, 76 g carbohydrate, 22 g protein, 629 mg sodium, 16 g fiber.

Edamame and Navy Bean Bowl

The edamame beans are a great source of protein and soy isoflavones, which may protect your heart and bones. The smooth texture of the edamame bean works well with the cheeses in this interesting dish.

- ¾ cup (168 g) shelled edamame beans
- ¼ cup (56 g) navy beans, rinsed and drained if canned
- ½ teaspoon (1.5 g) minced garlic
- 1 tablespoon feta cheese, crumbled
- 1 ounce (28 g) soft goat cheese, broken into small pieces
- 1½ tablespoons (25 ml) white balsamic vinegar
- 1 teaspoon flaxseed oil
- 2 teaspoons (2 g) basil, chopped

In a medium bowl, combine all ingredients and toss well.

Yield: 1 serving

Each will have: 405 calories, 20 g fat, 7.5 g saturated fat, 0 g trans fat, 21 mg cholesterol, 30 g carbohydrate, 27 g protein, 503 mg sodium, 11 g fiber.

Vegetarian Chili

Beans are a great source of fiber, which not only helps with digestion but can prevent blood-sugar levels from rising too rapidly after a meal. This can keep you full longer and help control your calorie intake! Balsamic vinegar is the secret ingredient in this recipe, enhancing the flavors.

- 1 teaspoon canola oil
- ½ cup (65 g) jicama, diced
- 2 tablespoons (20 g) onion, chopped
- 2 tablespoons (13 g) celery, chopped
- 2 tablespoons (15 g) grated carrots
- 2 tablespoons (15 g) green pepper, chopped
- ½ teaspoon garlic, minced
- 1 cup (235 ml) vegetable broth
- ½ cup (120 ml) water
- 1 tomato, chopped
- ½ cup (112 g) kidney beans, rinsed and drained
- ½ cup (112 g) pinto beans, rinsed and drained
- ½ teaspoon chili powder
- ½ teaspoon ground cumin
- 1 tablespoon (15 ml) balsamic vinegar

Heat canola oil in a skillet over medium heat. Add jicama, onions, celery, carrots, peppers, and garlic and sauté for 6 minutes. In a medium saucepan, combine sautéed vegetables, vegetable broth, water, tomato, kidney beans, pinto beans, chili powder, cumin, and vinegar. Bring just to a boil. Cover, reduce heat to low, and simmer for 15 minutes.

Yield: 1 serving

Each will have: 397 calories, 6 g fat, 1 g saturated fat, 0 g trans fat, 0 mg cholesterol, 72 g carbohydrate, 19 g protein, 544 mg sodium, 19 g fiber.

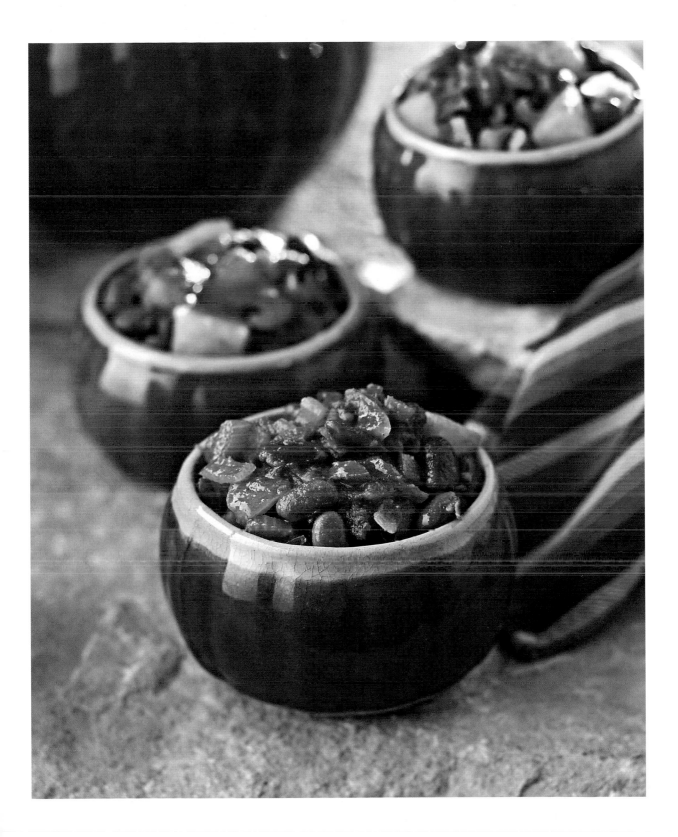

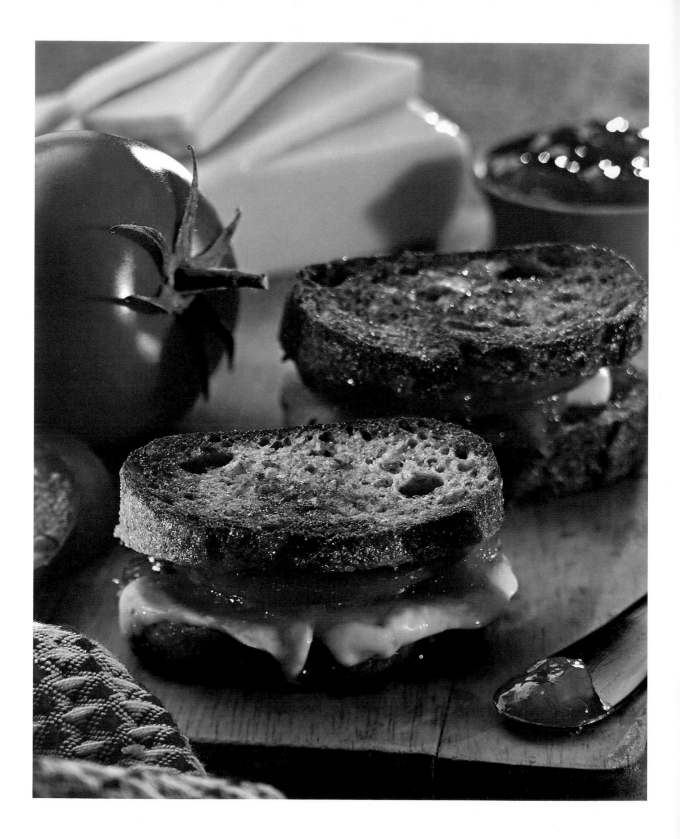

Soy Grilled Cheese

Low-fat soy cheese has no saturated fat and most brands provide up to 30 percent of your daily calcium needs. The insoluble fiber in the whole grain bread aids digestion by gently scraping the intestinal wall. Apricot lends a sweet surprise to this truly gourmet grilled cheese sandwich.

- Olive oil flavored cooking spray
- 2 slices whole-wheat French bread (about 2 ounces, or 60 g) or whole-wheat bread
- 2 teaspoons (10 ml) apricot preserves, divided
- 2 apricots, thinly sliced
- 4 teaspoons (20 g) light, trans-free margarine
- ½ tomato, sliced
- 2 slices soy cheese (mozzarella flavor works well)

Generously spray a skillet with cooking spray and heat over medium. Spread 1 side of each slice of bread with 2 teaspoons (10 ml) margarine and the other side with 1 teaspoon apricot preserves. Place slice of bread margarine side down in skillet, preserves-side facing up. Top with the apricots, tomato, cheese, and remaining slice of bread (preserves-side down), and grill on each side for 3 to 4 minutes or until golden brown.

Yield: 1 serving

Each will have: 269 calories, 5 g fat, 0 g saturated fat, 0 g trans fat, 0 mg cholesterol, 44 g carbohydrate, 17 g protein, 508 mg sodium, 5.8 g fiber.

TIP: MAKE IT A MEAL

Serve with 1 cup (235 ml) low-fat buttermilk and 1 cup (145 g) blueberries.

With buttermilk and blueberries, each will have: 450 calories, 8 g fat, 1.5 g saturated fat, 0 g trans fat, 10 mg cholesterol, 76 g carbohydrate, 26 g protein, 767 mg sodium, 9.3 g fiber.

Tuna and White Bean Pasta

Look for chunk light tuna since it has less mercury than other varieties of tuna. Just a half cup of white beans provide over 9 grams of lean protein, important for building your immune response when faced with an infection. This is a surprisingly savory, filling one-dish meal everyone in the family will love.

- ½ cup (112 g) canned white beans, rinsed and drained
- 3 ounces (85 g) chunk light tuna
- 1 tablespoon (15 ml) white vinegar
- 1 tablespoon (15 ml) lime juice
- 1 teaspoon olive oil
- 1 teaspoon capers, drained
- 2 teaspoons (7 g) red onion, finely chopped
- ½ cup (25 g) cooked whole-wheat pasta, any shape (rotini works well)

In a medium bowl, combine all ingredients and toss well.

Yield: 1 serving

Each will have: 448 calories, 15 g fat, 1.2 g saturated fat, 0 g trans fat, 45 mg cholesterol, 47 g carbohydrate, 33 g protein, 469 mg sodium, 8.4 g fiber.

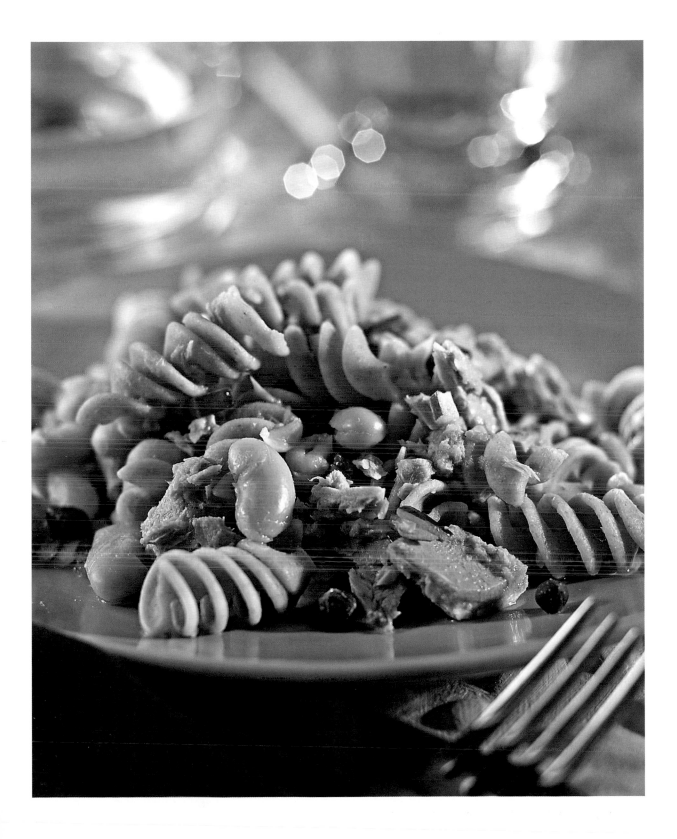

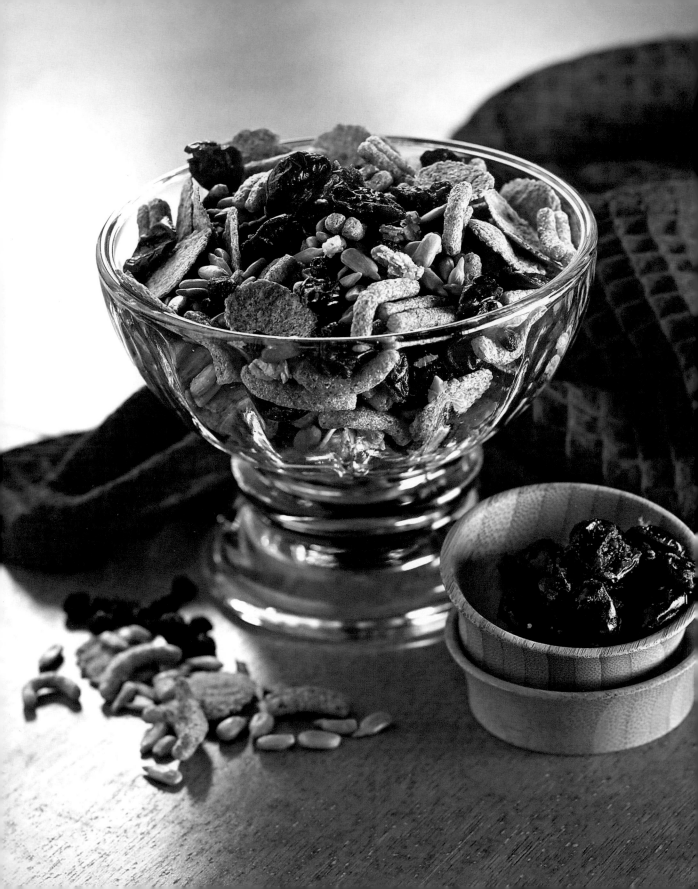

SNACKS

Sunflower Graham Yogurt

One cup of low-fat yogurt provides over 400 mg of calcium, even more than a cup of milk. Yogurt is also a great source of lean protein, a critical part of actin and myosin, which control proper mechanical function of your muscles. The nutty crunch of sunflower seeds makes this snack satisfying enough to get you through that afternoon slump.

- 4 ounces (115 g) low-fat plain yogurt
- 1 teaspoon (5 ml) agave nectar or honey
- 2 teaspoons (10 g) sunflower seeds, shelled
- 1 graham cracker, plain (one 2½ x 5-inch, or 6.4 x 12.7-cm, rectangle)

Drizzle yogurt with the agave nectar, top with the sunflower seeds, and crumble the cracker into the yogurt.

Yield: 1 serving

Each will have: 182 calories, 6 g fat, 1.6 g saturated fat, 0 g trans fat, 7 mg cholesterol, 25 g carbohydrate, 8 g protein, 186 mg sodium, 0.9 g fiber.

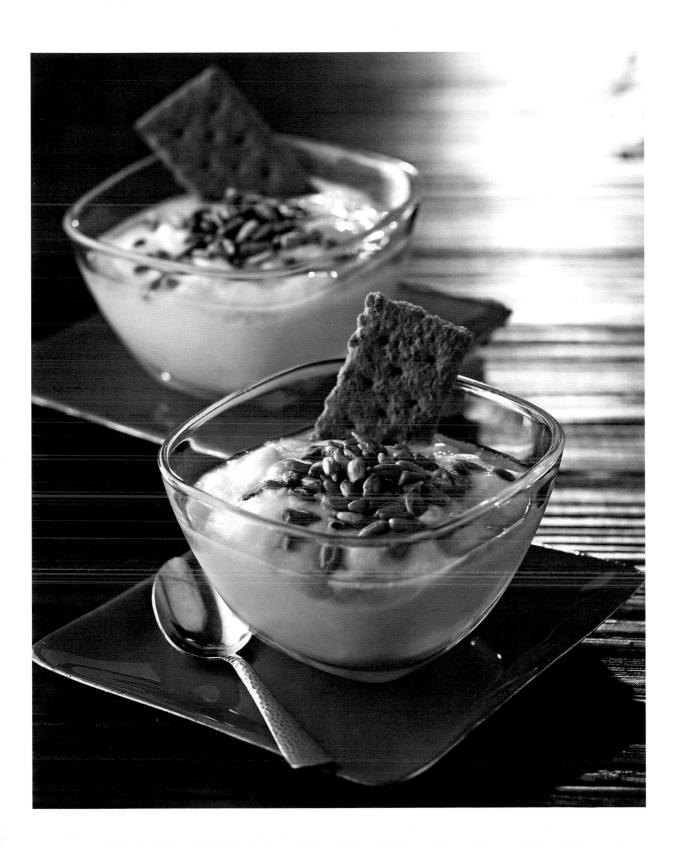

Maple Nut Oatmeal

Oats contain a special type of fiber known as beta glucan, which is very helpful for lowering your blood cholesterol level. The pecans add 2 grams of monounsaturated fats, which help to raise your HDL, or good cholesterol level.

- ½ cup (40 g) oatmeal, dry
- 1 cup (235 ml) water
- ¼ teaspoon maple extract
- 2 teaspoons (6 g) pecans, chopped

Make oatmeal with water according to package directions. Stir in maple extract and pecans.

Yield: 1 serving

Each will have: 187 calories, 6 g fat, 0.7 g saturated fat, 0 g trans fat, 0 mg cholesterol, 28 g carbohydrate, 6 g protein, 163 mg sodium, 4.4 g fiber.

Kiwi-Strawberry Cereal

This dish provides over 100 percent of your vitamin C, which has many health benefits, including reducing your risk for stroke.

- ½ cup (25 g) shredded-wheat cereal
- 4 ounces (115 g) low-fat fruit-flavored yogurt
- 1 kiwi, sliced
- 2 tablespoons (19 g) dried strawberries

In a bowl, combine cereal with yogurt and stir to blend well. Top with kiwi and strawberries.

Yield: 1 serving

Each will have: 282 calories, 2.6 g fat, 1 g saturated fat, 0 g trans fat, 10 mg cholesterol, 60 g carbohydrate, 8 g protein, 80 mg sodium, 6.5 g fiber.

Berry Flax Yogurt

Any type of berry you choose for this dish is rich in antioxidants, which are important for helping reduce your risk of cancer and heart disease. The alpha linolenic acid (ALA) in flax seeds is essential for producing anti-inflammatory molecules called prostaglandins.

- 4 ounces (115 g) low-fat plain yogurt
- ½ cup (72 g) blackberries
- 1 tablespoon (7 g) ground flaxseed

Top yogurt with berries and flaxseed.

Yield: 1 serving

Each will have: 140 calories, 5 g fat, 1.4 g saturated fat, 0 g trans fat, 7 mg cholesterol, 17 g carbohydrate, 8 g protein, 82 mg sodium, 6 g fiber.

Peach Yogurt

The peach is rich in soluble fiber which can reduce the symptoms of irritable bowel syndrome. The yogurt is a good source of iodine, which is stored and used by your thyroid gland to help produce hormones that help regulate growth and development as well as reproduction.

- 1 peach, thinly sliced
- 4 ounces (115 g) low-fat vanilla yogurt

Top yogurt with sliced peach.

Yield: 1 serving

Each will have: 169 calories, 2 g fat, 1.5 g saturated fat, 0 g trans fat, 10 mg cholesterol, 33 g carbohydrate, 7 g protein, 70 mg sodium, 2.3 g fiber.

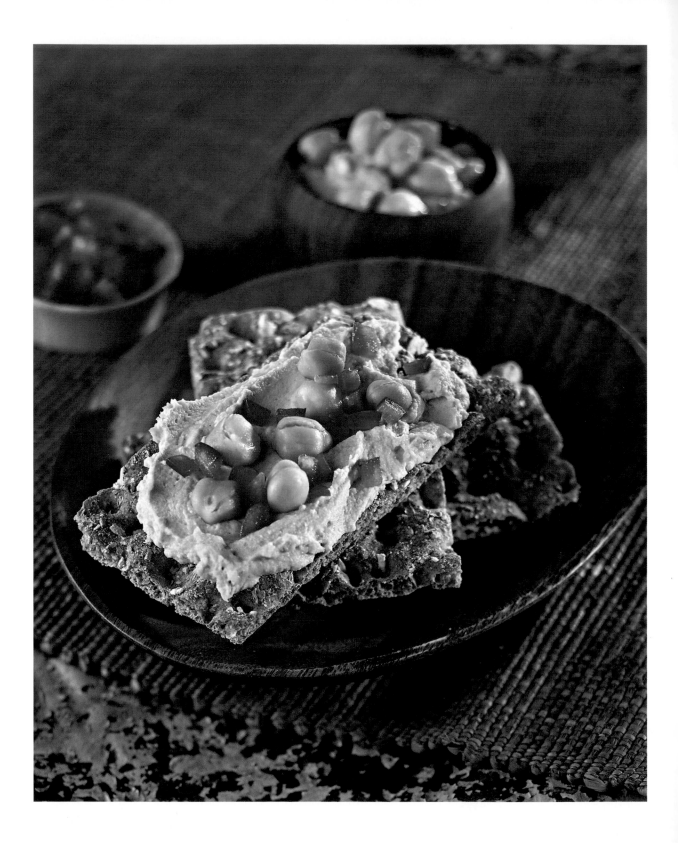

Garbanzo and Sweet Bell Pepper Crackers

Mediterranean flavors blend for a cracker you can sink your teeth into. When you choose a whole grain, high fiber cracker over a refined white flour cracker, you add up to 4 grams of fiber—and digestive help—to your snack!

- 2 whole-wheat crackers, such as Wasa Multi Grain crispbread
- 2 tablespoons (28 g) hummus
- ⅛ teaspoon paprika
- 2 tablespoons (30 g) garbanzo beans
- 2 teaspoons (5 g) bell pepper, finely chopped

Spread each cracker with half the hummus and garbanzo beans and top each with half the bell pepper. Sprinkle the tops with paprika.

Yield: 1 serving

Each will have: 177 calories, 3 g fat, 0 g saturated fat, 0 g trans fat, 7 mg cholesterol, 32 g carbohydrate, 7 g protein, 380 mg sodium, 6 g fiber.

Nutty Oat Muffin

Look for oat bran English muffins to provide soluble fiber to help lower your blood cholesterol level. The walnuts and the flax seeds are rich in alpha linolenic acid (ALA), which is good for reducing your risk for heart disease. You'll love this sweet and nutty combination.

- 1 oat bran English muffin
- 2 teaspoons (10 ml) agave nectar or honey
- 4 teaspoons (11 g) walnuts, chopped
- 2 teaspoons (5 g) ground flaxseed

Toast the English muffin. Top each half with half the agave nectar, walnuts, and flaxseed.

Yield: 2 servings

Each will have: 123 calories, 4 g fat, 0.5 g saturated fat, 0 g trans fat, 0 mg cholesterol, 20 g carbohydrate, 3 g protein, 106 mg sodium, 2.2 g fiber.

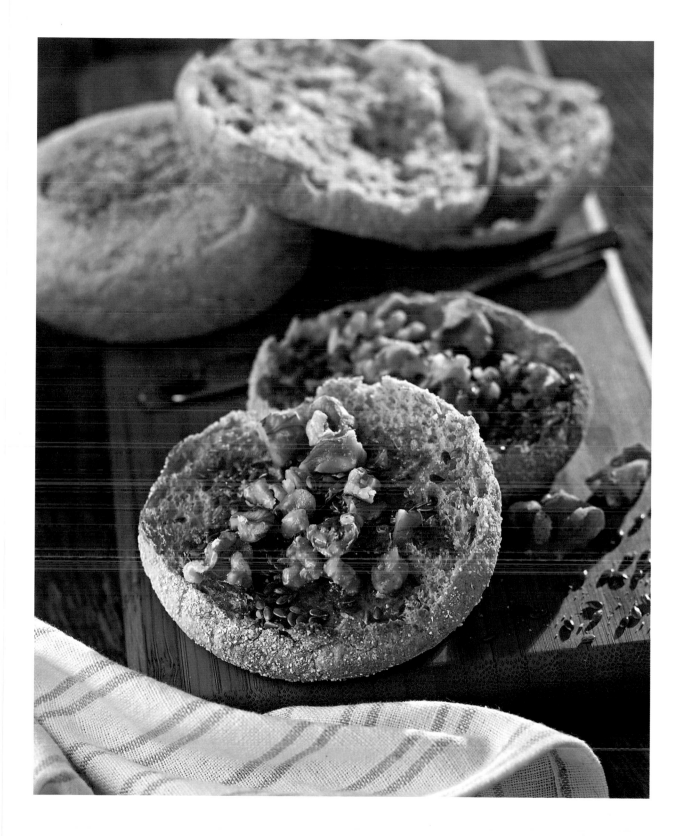

Tasty Trail Mix

A spoonful of dried blueberries provides over 1 gram of dietary fiber, higher than most dried fruits. Most high fiber, whole grain cereals pack 4 grams of fiber into a quarter cup making this snack a great way to add a little extra fiber to your day. This sweet and salty combination makes the perfect snack on-the-run.

- 1 tablespoon (9 g) dried cranberries
- 1 tablespoon (9 g) dried blueberries
- 1 tablespoon (14 g) sunflower seeds, shelled
- ¼ cup (13 g) whole-grain, high-fiber cereal

Combine all ingredients and store in a resealable plastic bag.

Yield: 1 serving

Each will have: 149 calories, 4 g fat, 0.4 g saturated fat, 0 g trans fat, 0 mg cholesterol, 29 g carbohydrate, 3 g protein, 97 mg sodium, 6.3 g fiber.

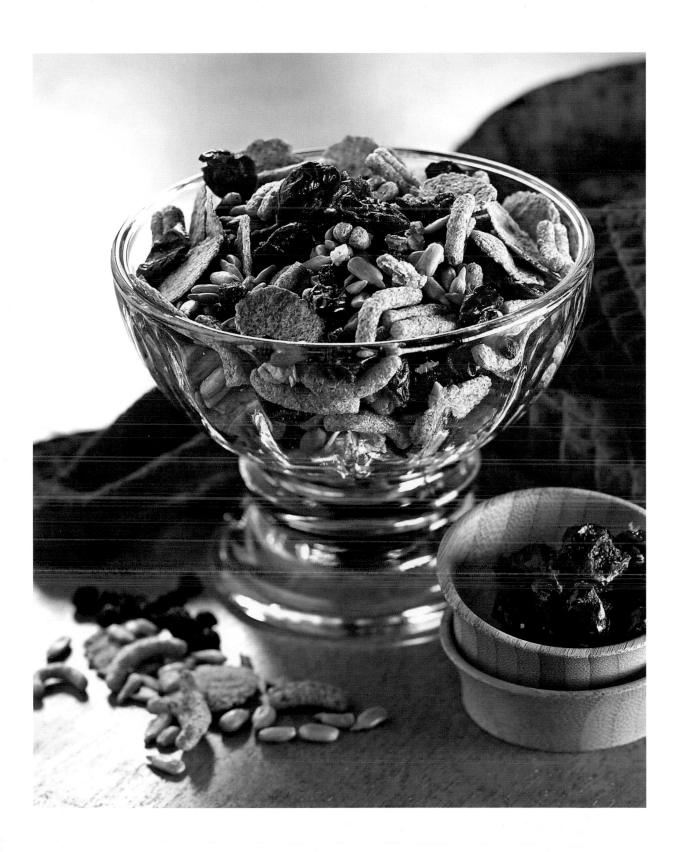

Tart Peach and Tomato Salsa

The peach and tomato combine to give you one quarter of your daily need of vitamin A, which is important for healthy skin and hair. A sweet and sour salsa with such a surprising combination of tastes, you'll want to make it for your next gathering.

- 2 tablespoons (20 g) chopped red onion
- 1 peach, diced
- 2 tomatoes, chopped
- 1 tablespoon (1 g) fresh cilantro, chopped
- 2 teaspoons (10 ml) lime juice
- 1 teaspoon flaxseed oil
- 4 whole-wheat crackers, such as Wasa Multi Grain crispbread

Combine all ingredients and scoop salsa with crackers.

Yield: 2 servings

Each will have: 165 calories, 3 g fat, 0.3 g saturated fat, 0 g trans fat, 0 mg cholesterol, 33 g carbohydrate, 9 g protein, 167 mg sodium, 6.7 g fiber.

Italian Bagel

A little bit of cheese goes a long way, providing 200 milligrams of calcium, about 20 percent of your daily value. Tomato sauce is rich in the antioxidant lycopene, which offers protection against stroke. Let the cheese melt for a minute for genuine pizza look and taste.

- 1 oat bran bagel, toasted
- 2 tablespoons (30 ml) pasta sauce
- 4 tablespoons (30 g) shredded mozzarella cheese
- 2 tablespoons (19 g) pineapple chunks, fresh, or canned in juice and drained

Preheat the oven to 200°F (90°C, or below gas mark ½). To assemble the bagel, top each half with half the sauce, cheese, and pineapple. Place on a baking sheet and bake until the cheese just begins to melt, about 4 to 5 minutes.

Yield: 1 serving

Each will have: 294 calories, 7 g fat, 3 g saturated fat, 0 g trans fat, 15 mg cholesterol, 45 g carbohydrate, 15 g protein, 627 mg sodium, 4 g fiber.

Berry Roll Up

Look for high fiber, whole grain wraps, which will save you a few calories and get some insoluble fiber to help fill you up and keep your digestive system moving along. A creamy, smooth, filling treat. Substitute your favorite berries for variety.

- 1 whole-wheat soft tortilla, such as Flatout Multi-Grain
- 4 ounces (115 g) low-fat fruit-flavored yogurt
- ½ cup (73 g) blueberries

Spread tortilla with yogurt and top with blueberries; roll up to eat.

Yield: 1 serving

Each will have: 251 calories, 5 g fat, 1 g saturated fat, 0 g trans fat, 5 mg cholesterol, 47 g carbohydrate, 15 g protein, 445 mg sodium, 9.7 g fiber.

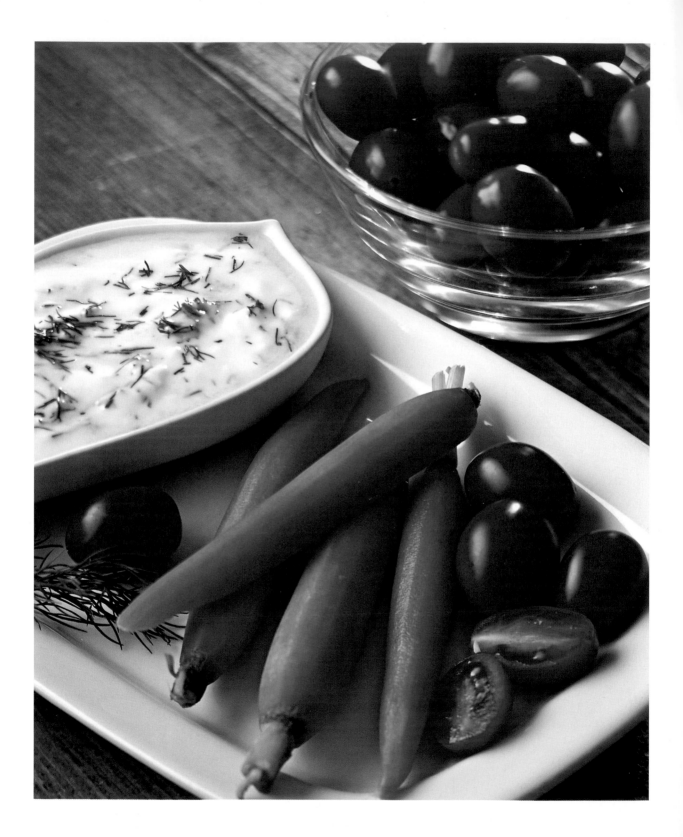

Savory Vegetable Dip

Low-fat yogurt is a great choice for making your dip because it's rich in calcium, phosphorus, and magnesium, three minerals that help manage blood pressure. This dip is so tasty that whenever you whip up a batch you'll be searching for more vegetables to dip.

- 4 ounces (115 g) low-fat plain yogurt
- ½ teaspoon dill
- 2 teaspoons (10 ml) lime juice
- ½ teaspoon flaxseed oil
- ⅛ teaspoon white horseradish sauce
- 2 tablespoons (30 g) chopped scallions
- 5 baby carrots
- 5 grape tomatoes
- 1 whole-wheat cracker, such as Wasa Multi Grain crispbread

In a bowl combine yogurt, dill, lime juice, horseradish, scallions, and flaxseed oil. Dip carrots, tomatoes, and crackers in yogurt dip.

Yield: 1 serving

Each will have: 178 calories, 4 g fat, 1.4 g saturated fat, 0 g trans fat, 9 mg cholesterol, 27 g carbohydrate, 9 g protein, 199 mg sodium, 4 g fiber.

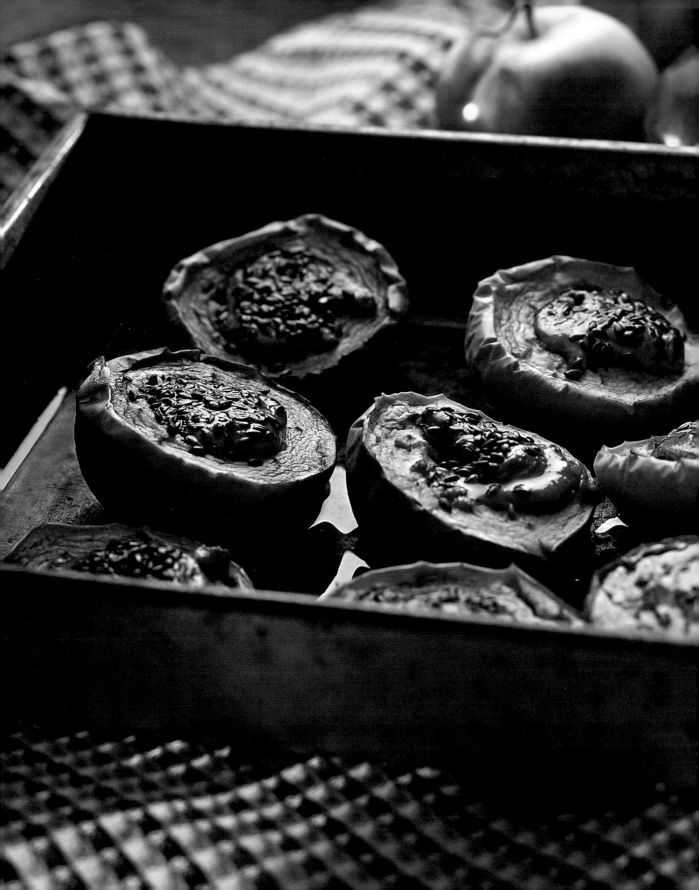

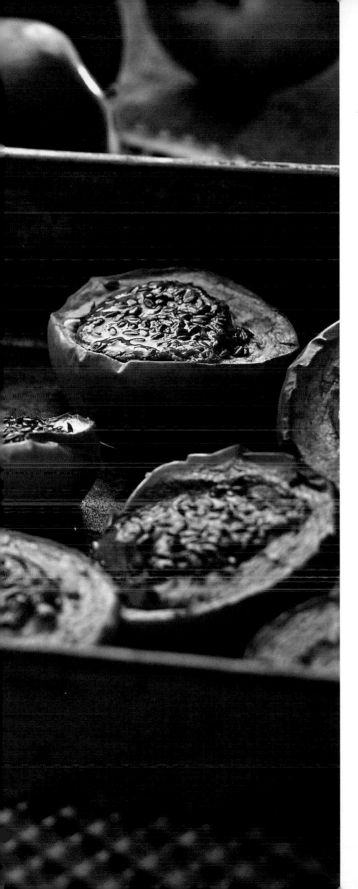

Baked Apple with Peanut Butter and Flax

Peanut butter provides mostly heart healthy monounsaturated fats. Check the ingredients list on your peanut butter label and choose one without partially hydrogenated oils to eliminate trans fats, which are linked to increased cholesterol levels and decreased HDL levels. Baking the apple gives it a mild flavor that will remind you of apple pie.

- 1 apple, sliced in half and cored
- 2 teaspoons (10 g) peanut butter
- 2 teaspoons (5 g) ground flaxseed

Preheat the oven to 375°F (190°C, or gas mark 5). Fill a small baking dish or roasting pan with ½ inch (1.3 cm) of water. Add the apple halves and bake for 30 minutes. Spread each apple half with half the peanut butter and ground flaxseed.

Yield: 1 serving

Each will have: 159 calories, 8 g fat, 1.3 g saturated fat, 0 g trans fat, 0 mg cholesterol, 24 g carbohydrate, 7 g protein, 52 mg sodium, 5 g fiber.

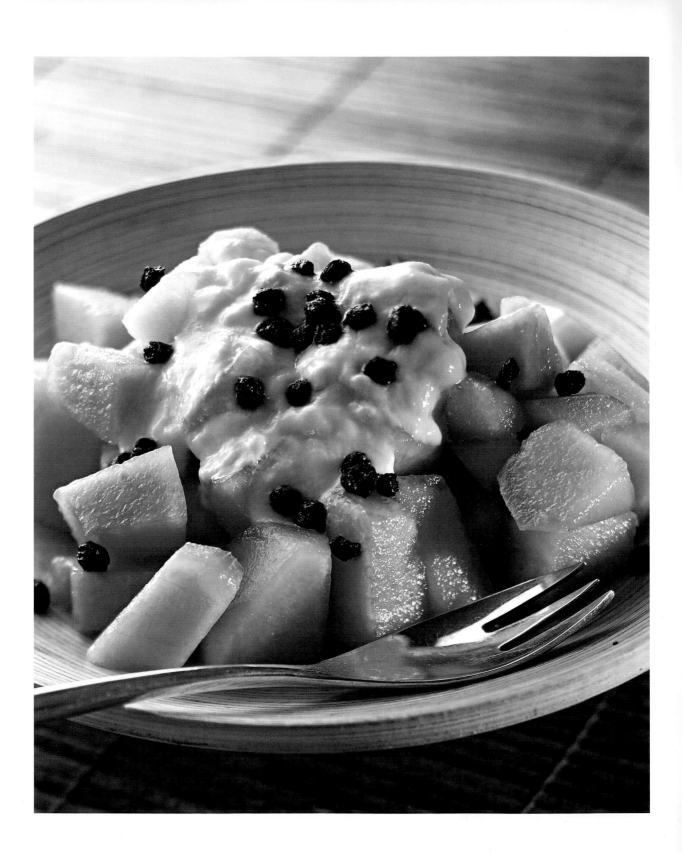

Fruit Salad Tossed with Yogurt Dressing

Honeydew melon is rich in potassium, a mineral that works with sodium to help regulate fluid balance in the body. Cantaloupe provides over 80 percent of your daily value of vitamin A, a fat-soluble vitamin that's important for eye health.

- 2 ounces (60 g) low-fat fruit-flavored yogurt
- ⅛ teaspoon pure vanilla extract
- ¾ cup (116 g) cantaloupe, cubed
- ¾ cup (116 g) honeydew, cubed
- 1 tablespoon (9 g) dried blueberries

Combine yogurt and vanilla extract; toss together with cantaloupe and honeydew. Sprinkle with dried blueberries.

Yield: 1 serving

Each will have: 238 calories, 2 g fat, 1 g saturated fat, 0 g trans fat, 10 mg cholesterol, 50 g carbohydrate, 7 g protein, 119 mg sodium, 3 g fiber.

Cranberry Oatmeal Tart

Cranberries contain quinic acid, which is not digested by the body and provides a beneficial effect in your kidneys to prevent kidney stone formation. Bring this recipe to your next gathering and you'll be the hit of the party.

For the pastry:

- Cooking spray
- ½ cup (60 g) whole-wheat pastry flour
- ⅛ teaspoon salt
- 2 teaspoons (9 g) granulated sugar
- 3 tablespoons (42 g) light, trans-fat-free margarine
- 3 tablespoons (15 g) rolled oats
- 2 tablespoons (30 ml) cold water

For the filling:

- ½ cup (55 g) fresh cranberries
- 1 tablespoon (13 g) granulated sugar
- 1 egg white
- ⅛ teaspoon pure vanilla extract

Preheat the oven to 425°F (220°C, or gas mark 7). Lightly spray the bottoms of a muffin tin with cooking spray.

To make the pastry, in a medium bowl, combine whole-wheat pastry flour with salt and sugar. Use a fork to mix margarine into the flour mixture until it resembles coarse crumbs. Add rolled oats and mix lightly with your fingers. Add water a little at a time until you can form the mixture into a ball. Divide pastry into four portions and press into the bottoms only of 4 muffin cups.

Combine filling ingredients and spoon 1½ tablespoons (25 ml) into a depression made into each pastry shell. Bake for 10 to 12 minutes.

Yield: 4 servings

Each will have: 128 calories, 4 g fat, 0.8 g saturated fat, 0 g trans fat, 0 mg cholesterol, 20 g carbohydrate, 3 g protein, 151 mg sodium, 2.5 g fiber.

Buttermilk and English Muffin

Look for oat bran English muffins with at least three grams of fiber to get the benefit of both soluble and insoluble fiber which both help digestion.

- ½ oat bran English muffin
- 2 teaspoons (10 g) almond butter
- 1 cup (235 ml) low-fat buttermilk

Toast the English muffin, top with almond butter. Serve with buttermilk to drink.

Yield: 1 serving

Each will have: 286 calories, 9 g fat, 2.4 g saturated fat, 0 g trans fat, 10 mg cholesterol, 40 g carbohydrate, 14 g protcin, 515 mg sodium, 2.4 g fiber.

Waffle with Banana

Whole-grain waffles are a treat any time of day. Pair with a different fruit next time for variety.

- 1 whole-grain waffle
- 2 ounces (60 g) low-fat fruit-flavored yogurt
- 1 banana, thinly sliced

Toast the waffle and spread with the yogurt. Slice the banana over the top.

Yield: 1 serving

Each will have: 245 calories, 3 g fat, 0.6 g saturated fat, 0 g trans fat, 5 mg cholesterol, 53 g carbohydrate, 8 g protein, 204 mg sodium, 6 g fiber.

Green Tomatoes with Flatbread Points

Two green tomatoes have nearly three grams of fiber, which eases the passage of food and waste through your intestines. They are also full of vitamin A, which aids in regulating cell differentiation, allowing your cells to take on new roles in your body. The green tomatoes in this dish lend a unique flair to this salsa verde.

- Cooking spray
- 2 green tomatoes, chopped (may substitute red tomatoes)
- 1 teaspoon fresh cilantro
- 1 teaspoon flaxseed oil
- 2 teaspoons (10 ml) white balsamic vinegar
- 1 whole-wheat soft tortilla, such as Flatout Multi-Grain

Preheat the oven to 350°F (180°C, or gas mark 4). Coat a baking sheet with cooking spray; place chopped tomatoes on a baking sheet and bake for 17 minutes. Turn the heat down to 200°F (90°C, or below gas mark ½), place the tortilla on the center rack, and bake for 5 minutes. Break or slice into 4 triangle-shaped sections.

Combine tomatoes, cilantro, flaxseed oil, and vinegar and scoop the mixture with the tortilla pieces.

Yield: 1 serving

Each will have: 200 calories, 8 g fat, 0.5 g saturated fat, 0 g trans fat, 0 mg cholesterol, 30 g carbohydrate, 12 g protein, 412 mg sodium, 11 g fiber.

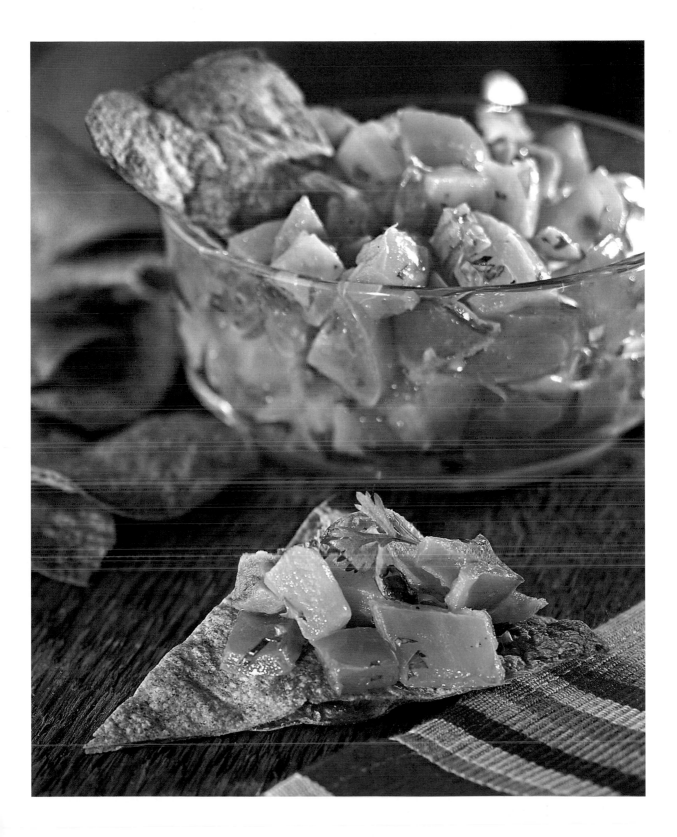

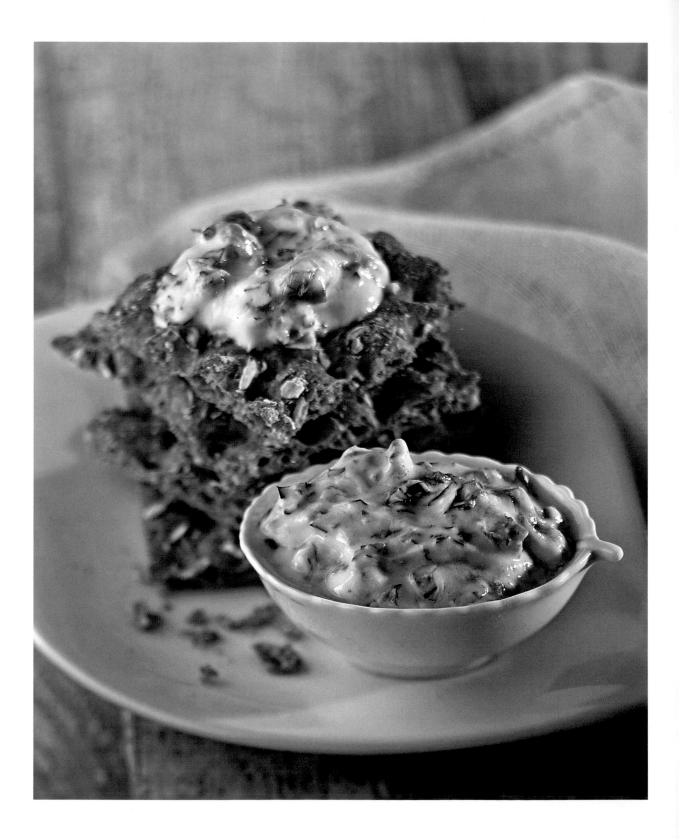

Sun-Dried Tomato Topping

Sun-dried tomatoes are packed with vitamin C. Two tablespoons provide 25 percent of your daily value of this antioxidant vitamin. The tomato and basil are fresh additions to this creamy, tasty spread.

- 2 tablespoons (14 g) sun-dried tomatoes packed in oil, drained and chopped
- 3 ounces (85 g) low-fat plain yogurt
- 1 teaspoon fresh basil, chopped
- 1 teaspoon flaxseed oil
- 2 whole-wheat crackers, such as Wasa Multi-Grain crispbread

Combine sun-dried tomatoes, yogurt, basil, and flaxseed oil. Spread over the crackers.

Yield: 1 serving

Each will have: 213 calories, 8 g fat, 1.5 g saturated fat, 0 g trans fat, 5 mg cholesterol, 29 g carbohydrate, 9 g protein, 256 mg sodium, 4.8 g fiber.

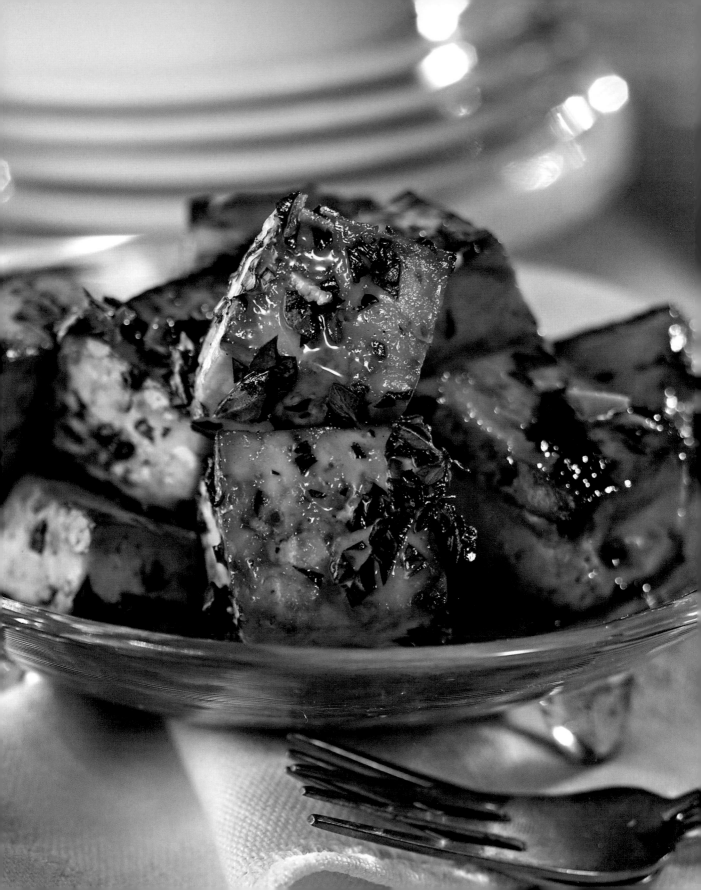

DINNERS

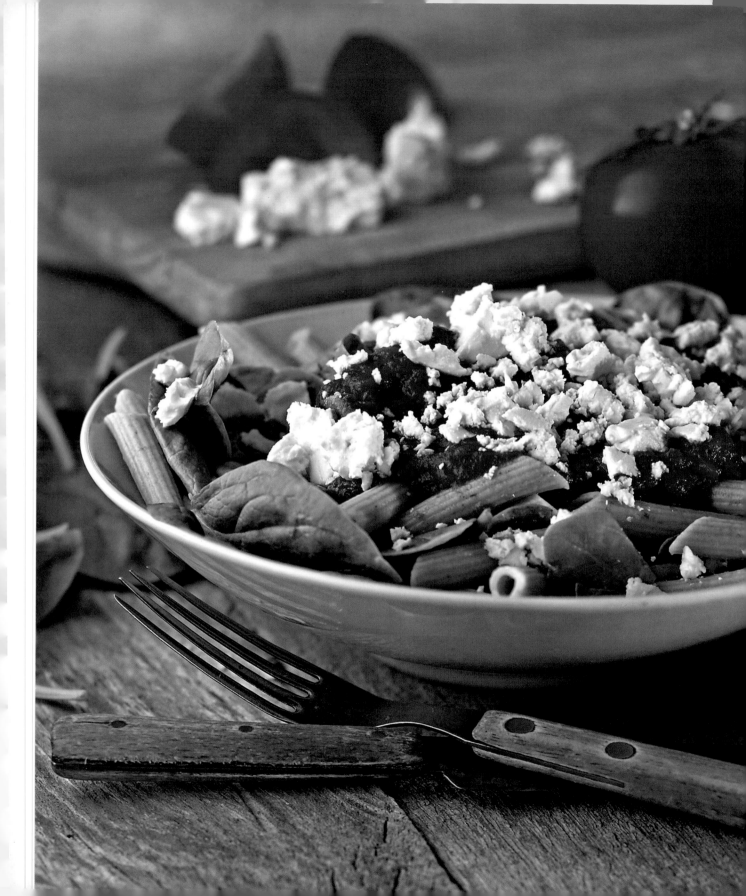

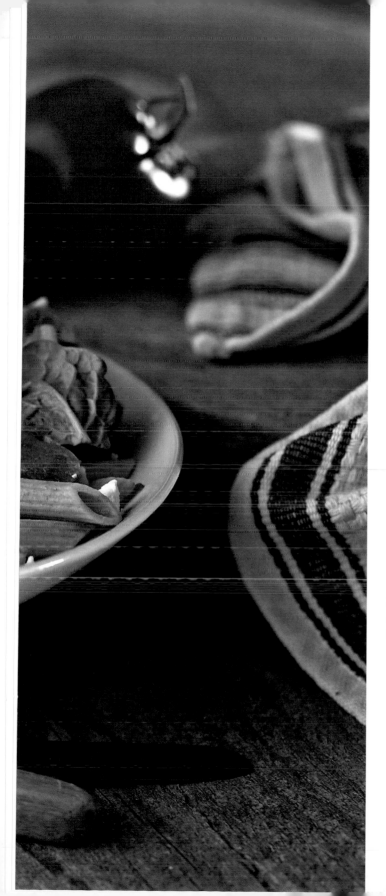

Pasta with Spinach

Two cups of spinach provides you with 60 mg of calcium, and recent research shows that calcium from green vegetables is bioavailable, which means it's very easy for your body to absorb during digestion. Try a spicy pasta sauce, such as one spiked with cayenne pepper, as a complement to the spinach and feta.

- ¾ cup (112 g) dry whole-wheat pasta, any shape (penne works well)
- ¾ cup (175 ml) spaghetti sauce
- 2 cups (40 g) fresh spinach leaves
- ¼ cup (38 g) reduced-fat feta cheese

Prepare pasta according to package directions. In a bowl, combine cooked pasta, sauce, spinach, and feta cheese. Heat in microwave for 45 seconds, stir, and heat for another 30 seconds.

Yield: 1 serving

Each will have: 477 calories, 12 g fat, 5.8 g saturated fat, 0 g trans fat, 33 mg cholesterol, 73 g carbohydrate, 22 g protein, 922 mg sodium, 11 g fiber.

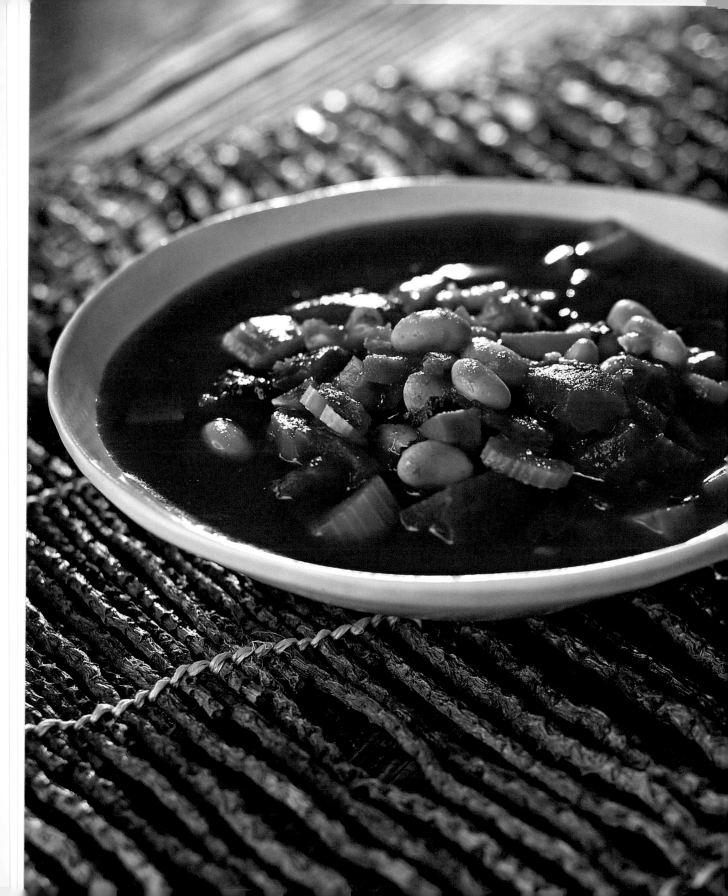

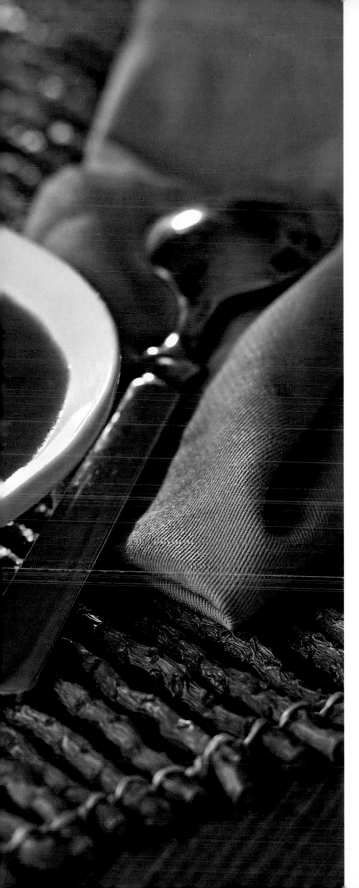

Minestrone Soup

Assemble this simple soup in less than 30 minutes for a hearty one-dish, digestion-friendly meal. Choose a low sodium broth for all of your soups and you can save up to 900 mg sodium per one cup serving!

- 2 teaspoons (10 ml) olive oil
- ½ cup (65 g) chopped carrots
- ½ cup (80 g) chopped onion
- ½ cup (50 g) chopped celery
- 2 teaspoons (6 g) minced garlic
- 1 tablespoon (2.5 g) chopped fresh basil
- 1 cup (235 ml) low-sodium vegetable broth
- 1 cup (235 ml) water
- 16 ounces (455 g) canned Great Northern beans, rinsed and drained
- 1 cup (235 ml) pasta sauce
- 1 cup (180 g) chopped tomatoes

Heat the olive oil in a large skillet over medium heat. Add the carrots, onion, celery, garlic, and basil and sauté until onion is translucent. Reduce heat to low, add the remaining ingredients, and simmer for 20 minutes.

Yield: 2 servings

Each will have: 423 calories, 7 g fat, 0.9 g saturated fat, 0 g trans fat, 0 mg cholesterol, 68 g carbohydrate, 23 g protein, 388 mg sodium, 17 g fiber.

Salmon with Cucumber Pasta

When you choose whole-wheat instead of white-flour pasta, you add almost three grams of fiber to your meal to bolster digestion. The citrus flavors combine to season the salmon without much added fat, and the cucumber makes a satisfying crunch with each bite.

- ½ cup (75 g) whole-wheat pasta, dry
- 3 ounces (85 g) salmon
- 1 teaspoon (5 ml) lime juice
- 1 teaspoon (5 ml) lemon juice
- 1 teaspoon (5 ml) olive oil
- 1½ tablespoons (25 ml) white vinegar
- ½ small cucumber, chopped
- 1 tomato, chopped
- 1 teaspoon fresh dill, chopped
- ¼ teaspoon ground black pepper

Preheat the oven to 400°F (200°C, or gas mark 6). Cook pasta according to package directions; allow to cool in a large serving bowl at room temperature. Place salmon on a piece of aluminum foil and bake for 8 minutes or until salmon flakes easily with a fork. Flake salmon into small pieces over the top of the pasta. Add remaining ingredients and toss well to combine. Serve at room temperature or chilled.

Yield: 1 serving

Each will have: 434 calories, 15 g fat, 2.7 g saturated fat, 0 g trans fat, 50 mg cholesterol, 51 g carbohydrate, 30 g protein, 65 mg sodium, 6.8 g fiber.

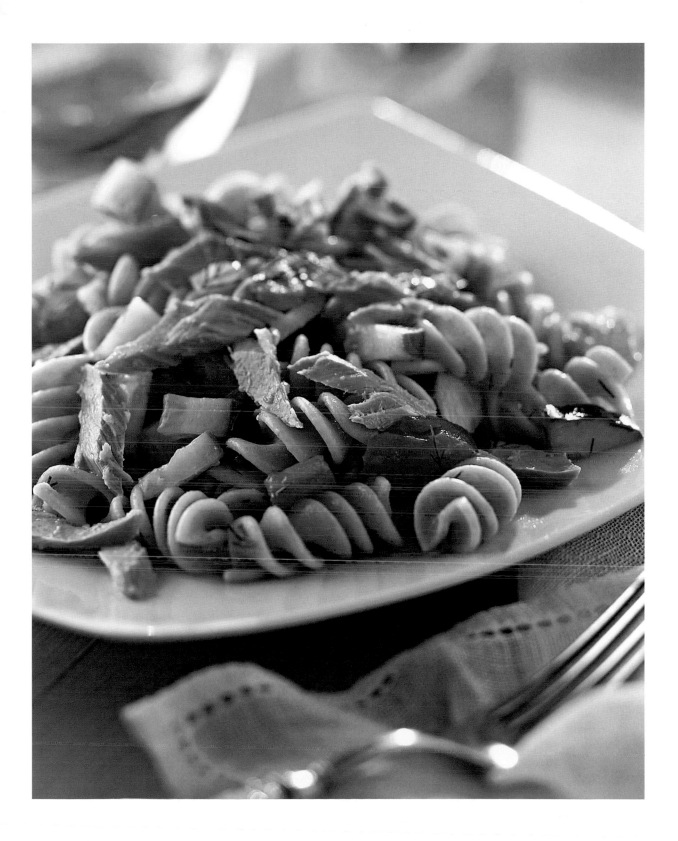

Pasta with Olive and Garlic Marinara Sauce

Garlic is a member of the lily or allium family and is rich in a variety of powerful sulfur-containing compounds including thiosulfinates. Studies show that thiosulfinates are good for managing triglyceride levels and an elevation of these blood fats is linked to increased risk for heart disease and diabetes. Fresh basil brings the flavors alive in this dish.

- ¾ cup (112 g) whole-wheat pasta, uncooked (angel hair works well)
- 1 teaspoon olive oil
- 1 teaspoon shallot, finely chopped
- 1 teaspoon garlic, minced
- ⅓ cup (80 ml) no-salt-added tomato paste
- 1 cup (235 ml) no-salt-added stewed tomatoes, undrained
- 2 tablespoons (30 ml) vegetable broth
- 2 tablespoons (12 g) black olives, sliced
- 2 teaspoons (2 g) basil, chopped
- 2 tablespoons (10 g) Parmesan cheese, grated

Prepare the pasta according to package directions; set aside. Heat the olive oil in a saucepan over medium heat. Add the shallot and garlic to the pan and sauté for 2 minutes. Add the tomato paste, stewed tomatoes, vegetable broth, olives, and basil and reduce heat to low. Simmer, covered, for 7 minutes. To serve, spoon sauce over pasta and top with parmesan cheese.

Yield: 1 serving

Each will have: 534 calories, 11 g fat, 2.9 g saturated fat, 0 g trans fat, 9 mg cholesterol, 96 g carbohydrate, 24 g protein, 453 mg sodium, 12.7 g fiber.

Kimchi

One cup of cabbage has 100 percent of your daily value of vitamin K, which helps blood to clot and secludes the damaged area from infection or injury to begin the healing process. This is a lower-sodium version of the favorite Korean fermented cabbage.

- 2 heads Chinese cabbage, Napa cabbage, or bok choy, shredded
- 1 tablespoon (18 g) sea salt, or non-iodized salt
- 10 scallions, thinly sliced, including green tops
- 2 to 3 cloves garlic, crushed
- 1 (1-inch, or 2.5-cm) piece ginger, finely chopped
- 1 onion, chopped
- 1 tablespoon (15 ml) kimchi sauce (available at Asian markets)
- 4 tablespoons (30 g) Korean chili powder or 3 tablespoons (23 g) Mexican chili powder
- 2 tablespoons (25 g) brown sugar

Place the cabbage in several large, clean plastic bags, such as resealable plastic bags. Sprinkle the salt onto your wet hands, then rub it into the cabbage pieces. Use your hands to squeeze as much water out of the cabbage as possible. Once finished, seal the bag and set aside on the counter for at least 5 to 6 hours.

Take the cabbage out of the salt solution and rinse it, then squeeze out the excess water. Place cabbage back in the resealable plastic bags. Add the scallions, garlic, ginger, and onion to the cabbage mixture and mix well. Add kimchi sauce, chili powder, and sugar, stirring well to combine. Lay the bag out on the counter for two days. The kimchi is ready when it's soft in consistency, but not too mushy, with a little crunchiness left in the larger pieces. After two days, store the kimchi in the refrigerator.

Yield: 10 servings

Each will have: 37 calories, 0.6 g fat, 0.1 g saturated fat, 0 g trans fat, 0 mg cholesterol, 8 g carbohydrate, 2 g protein, 738 mg sodium, 2.4 g fiber.

Halibut and Roasted Apricot Wild Rice

Wild rice is a whole-grain food, which takes a little longer to digest, keeping you full longer. Roasting apricots brings out a mild, sweet flavor that enhances the rice.

- ½ cup (80 g) wild rice, uncooked
- 4 ounces (115 g) halibut
- 1 teaspoon dill
- ½ teaspoon ground black pepper
- 1 teaspoon lemon juice
- Cooking spray
- 2 apricots, chopped

Prepare rice according to package directions. Preheat the oven to 400°F (200°C, or gas mark 6). Place the fish on a sturdy piece of aluminum foil, sprinkle with lemon juice, pepper, and dill, and bake for 7 to 8 minutes or until the fish flakes easily with a fork. Reduce heat to 350°F (180°C, or gas mark 4). Coat a baking sheet with cooking spray. Place the apricots on the sheet and bake for 20 to 22 minutes. Sprinkle apricots over the cooked rice and serve along with the fish.

Yield: 1 serving

Each will have: 441 calories, 4 g fat, 0.6 g saturated fat, 0 g trans fat, 46 mg cholesterol, 60 g carbohydrate, 41 g protein, 86 mg sodium, 5.8 g fiber.

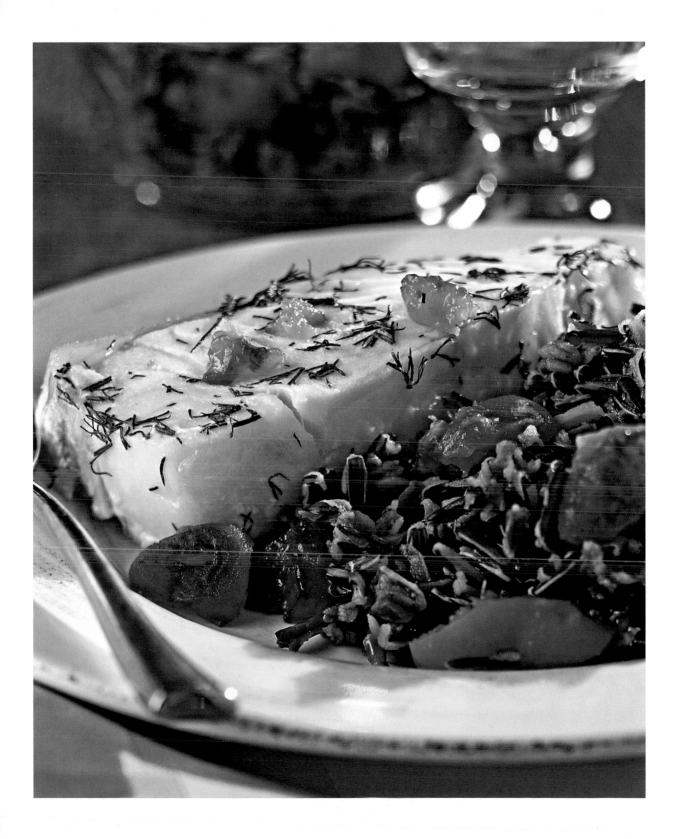

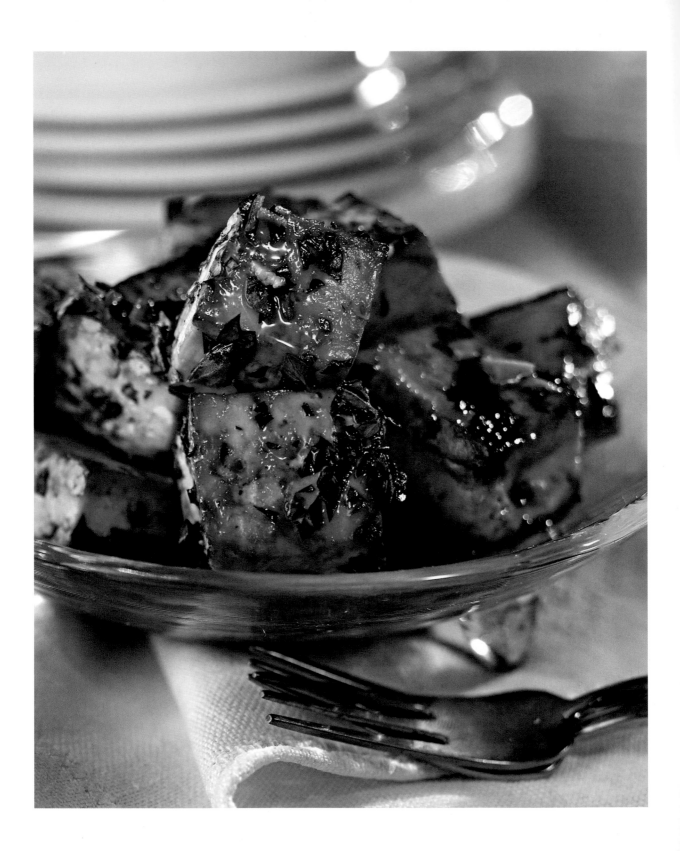

Lime Tamari Tofu Squares

Tofu is one of the rare sources of lean protein that includes fiber to facilitate digestive health.

- Cooking spray
- 2 tablespoons (30 ml) lime juice
- 1 tablespoon (15 ml) reduced-sodium tamari
- 2 teaspoons (10 ml) olive oil
- 2 teaspoons (2.5 g) fresh oregano
- 2 teaspoons (1.5 g) fresh thyme
- 2 teaspoons (2 g) fresh basil
- 1 teaspoon agave nectar
- 8 ounces (225 g) firm tofu, cut into squares

Preheat the oven to 375°F (190°C, or gas mark 5). Spray a 9 x 13-inch (22 x 33-cm) pan with cooking spray. In a large bowl, combine all ingredients except the tofu; stir well to combine. Add the tofu to the bowl and gently stir to coat the tofu. Allow to marinate in the bowl for 10 minutes. Lay tofu in prepared pan, being careful not to overlap the pieces, and bake for 15 minutes. Remove the pan from the oven and turn the tofu over; continue baking for 12 minutes. Pour any remaining marinade over the tofu to serve.

Yield: 2 servings

Each will have: 140 calories, 9 g fat, 1.6 g saturated fat, 0 g trans fat, 0 mg cholesterol, 7 g carbohydrate, 10 g protein, 365 mg sodium, 1 g fiber.

TIP: MAKE IT A MEAL

Sauté 1 cup (165 g) cooked brown rice and 1 cup (20 g) turnip greens with 1 teaspoon (5 ml) canola oil over medium heat, stirring frequently for 6 to 7 minutes. Serve tofu over rice mixture.

With rice and greens, each will have: 412 calories, 16 g fat, 2.6 g saturated fat, 0 g trans fat, 0 mg cholesterol, 55 g carbohydrate, 15 g protein, 383 mg sodium, 6 g fiber.

Apple Quinoa Salad

This gluten-free grain is a good source of fiber, to sustain digestion, and manganese, which activates enzymes that help your body use vitamin C. Quinoa is anything but bland when paired with sweet apple and crunchy celery.

For the salad:

- ⅓ cup (57 g) quinoa, dry
- 1 apple, chopped
- ½ cup (60 g) bell pepper, sliced
- 2 tablespoons (16 g) walnuts, chopped

For the dressing:

- 2 tablespoons (30 ml) apple juice
- 1 teaspoon reduced-sodium soy sauce
- 1 teaspoon agave nectar or honey
- ⅛ teaspoon curry powder
- ⅛ teaspoon cayenne pepper

Prepare quinoa according to package directions and set aside. To make the dressing, in a small bowl whisk together apple juice, soy sauce, agave nectar, curry powder, and cayenne pepper. Combine the quinoa, apple, pepper, and walnuts and toss with the dressing.

Yield: 1 serving

Each will have: 439 calories, 13 g fat, 1 g saturated fat, 0 g trans fat, 0 mg cholesterol, 74 g carbohydrate, 16 g protein, 210 mg sodium, 9.6 g fiber.

Japanese Swordfish and Greens

Turnip greens are packed with vitamins K, A, C, and folate, and linked to decreased risk of many diseases, including colon cancer and atherosclerosis.

- Cooking spray
- 1½ teaspoons reduced-sodium teriyaki sauce
- ½ teaspoon lemon zest
- ½ teaspoon garlic, minced
- 4 ounces (115 g) swordfish
- 1 teaspoon sesame oil
- 1 cup (20 g) turnip greens
- 1 teaspoon (2 g) ginger, chopped
- ¼ teaspoon ground black pepper

Preheat the oven to 375°F (190°C, or gas mark 5). Coat a baking dish with cooking spray. In a resealable plastic bag, combine teriyaki sauce, lemon zest, and garlic. Add the swordfish and marinate in the refrigerator for 10 minutes. Place swordfish in prepared baking dish and bake for 15 minutes or until fish flakes easily with a fork. Heat the oil in a skillet over medium heat. Add the turnip greens to the pan and season with ginger and pepper. Toss constantly until wilted and soft, about 4 minutes. Serve fish with the greens on the side.

Yield: 1 serving

Each will have: 208 calories, 9 g fat, 2 g saturated fat, 0 g trans fat, 44 mg cholesterol, 6 g carbohydrate, 24 g protein, 344 mg sodium, 1.8 g fiber.

TIP: MAKE IT A MEAL

Serve with ¾ cup (125 g) cooked brown rice tossed with ½ cup (77 g) pineapple chunks and ¼ teaspoon (1 ml) sesame oil.

With rice, pineapple, and oil, each will have: 452 calories, 12 g fat, 2.3 g saturated fat, 0 g trans fat, 44 mg cholesterol, 58 g carbohydrate, 27 g protein, 356 mg sodium, 5.4 g fiber.

Scallops and Rice

Scallops are a good source of vitamin B12, which is important for good cardiovascular health. A Dutch oven is a great addition to your kitchen. It allows you to cook dishes more slowly, really savoring the flavors.

- ½ cup (95 g) brown rice, dry
- ¼ cup (40 g) onion, chopped
- 1 garlic clove, minced
- 1 green bell pepper, chopped
- 1 (8-ounce, or 235-ml) can no-salt-added chopped tomatoes, undrained
- 1 teaspoon basil, chopped
- 2 teaspoons (10 ml) lemon juice
- 1 teaspoon thyme, chopped
- ½ teaspoon ground black pepper
- 1 teaspoon granulated sugar
- 1 teaspoon canola oil
- ⅛ teaspoon paprika
- 4 ounces (115 g) scallops

Prepare brown rice according to package directions; set aside. Preheat oven to 350°F (180°C, or gas mark 4). In a covered Dutch oven or casserole dish, combine onion, garlic, pepper, tomatoes (including liquid), basil, thyme, ground black pepper, sugar, oil, and paprika. Simmer for 20 minutes. Bring mixture to a boil, then add scallops and cook for 3 to 4 minutes. Serve scallops and vegetables over the brown rice.

Yield: 1 serving

Each will have: 466 calories, 7 g fat, 0.8 g saturated fat, 0 g trans fat, 37 mg cholesterol, 74 g carbohydrate, 28 g protein, 115 mg sodium, 10.4 g fiber.

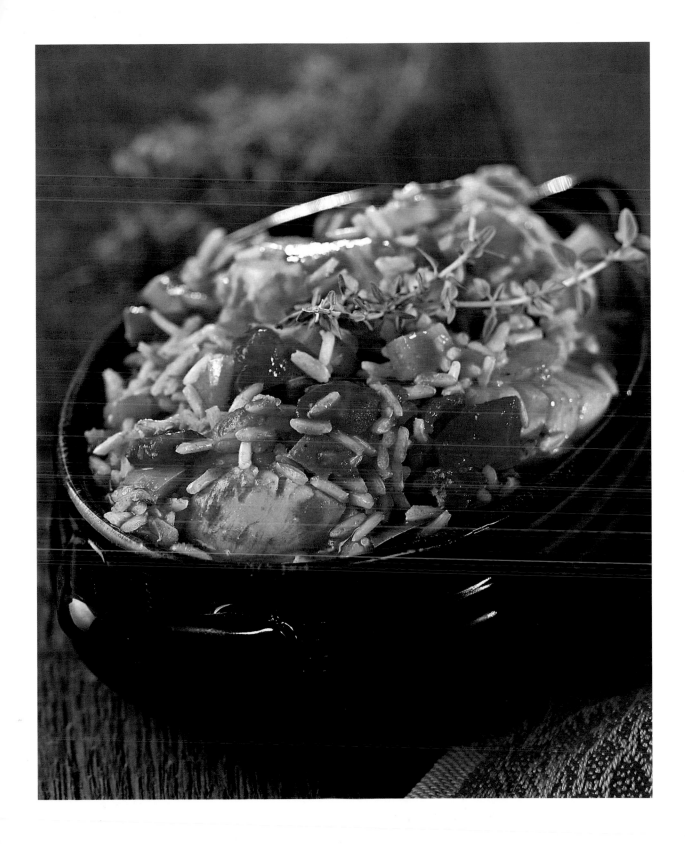

Index

Page numbers in *italics* indicate photographs.